26 (2-96) 0

ALSO BY MARY FISHER

Sleep with the Angels

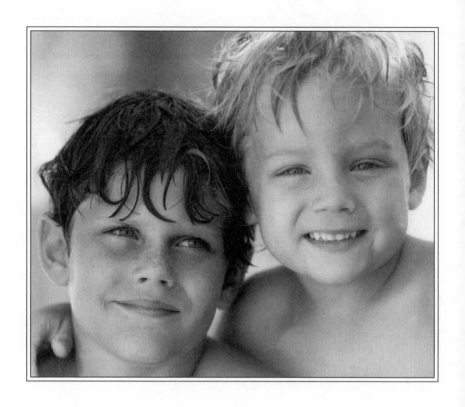

I'LL NOT GO QUIETLY

MARY

FISHER

SPEAKS

OUT

MARY FISHER

WITH AN INTRODUCTION BY KATIE COURIC

SCRIBNER

New York   London   Toronto   Sydney   Tokyo   Singapore

SCRIBNER
1230 Avenue of the Americas
New York, NY 10020

SCRIBNER and design are trademarks of Simon & Schuster Inc.

Designed by Jennifer Dossin

Manufactured in the United States of America
1 3 5 7 9 10 8 6 4 2
Poem beginning with "Your death blows a strange . . ." from A Grief Observed
by C. S. Lewis. Copyright © 1961 by N. W. Clerk. Reprinted by permission of
HarperCollins Publishers, Inc.

Photo credits: p. 97—Patti Cooney; pp. 4, 17, 25, 31, 45, 57, 71, 77, 85, 111,
121, 129, 149, 161, 175, 187, 199—Mary Fisher; p. 143—David Kennerly

Library of Congress Cataloging-in-Publication Data
Fisher, Mary 1948–
I'll not go quietly: Mary Fisher speaks out/by Mary Fisher.
p. cm.
1. AIDS (Disease) 2. AIDS (Disease)—United States. I. Title.
RC607.A26F55   1995
362.1'969792—dc20   95–6450
CIP
ISBN 0-684-80074-8

CONTENTS

ACKNOWLEDGMENTS

Jennifer Moyer first encouraged us to put public speeches and private photographs into book form. I remain in her debt.

Leigh Haber is the editor who brought us to Scribner. Ron Konecky, a world-class attorney, is always available when we need wise counsel. These two people simultaneously assembled contracts and manuscripts, making this book both possible and timely.

Katie Couric is extraordinary. She anchors what may be the most influential television program in history while retaining the common touch of a sister and the easy kindness we associate with a good neighbor. I've enjoyed her friendship since first we met—moments before we went on camera—and I'm grateful for her kind introduction to this collection.

Without my children, Max and Zachary, I'd lack the passion to speak out at all. My sons exhaust me in ways all young children exhaust their parents. But other parents will understand that they are also what motivates me to do what I'd otherwise never dream of doing.

And without Jim (A. James Heynen), there would be no book because there would be no speeches. I can picture my experience through a camera's lens, or in my studio. But until Jim arrived three years ago, I could never express it adequately in words. The gift he brought was himself: when he writes for me, he gives voice to my soul.

Some readers will be familiar with our first anthology of photographs and speeches, drawn from my early months in the AIDS community. It began with a letter to my children, which closed, as does each of their days, with me tucking them into bed and saying, "sleep with the angels." By comparison, this book—*I'll Not Go Quietly*—opens at the memorial service for their father.

I'm no less a mother now than I was a year or two ago. But I'm more a veteran in the AIDS war. I've seen the brutal stigma, the terror, the anger, the fear. I've tasted the dying. Like veterans of other wars, I've stood amid the carnage and counted the casualties. Early on, I could name each person whom I'd lost. But I can't name them all anymore. I can only grieve them, one by one.

It's to them, my fellow pilgrims no longer marching with us, that I dedicate this book. I feel their absence as if they've gone away, even though I believe they've only gone ahead. Their memory deserves more than a few photographs and speeches. Yet it's a beginning, to dedicate to them a book and a solemn promise: I'll not go quietly.

Valentine's Day, 1995

INTRODUCTION

There is nothing like death looming on the horizon to wipe away pretense. Nothing like the knowledge that one's life will end before some grand design or intended heavenly blueprint, to destroy any false pleasantries or superficial civilities. Something tells me Mary Fisher never had much patience for any of that, that she has always been disarmingly REAL. But ever since she was diagnosed with the AIDS virus, she has made it painfully clear that she is here for a reason. To educate, to enlighten, to inform, to talk honestly about herself and the community she represents.

In July 1991, Mary Fisher received a telephone call from her ex-husband, Brian Campbell. Mary and Brian had moved to Florida as newlyweds; their marriage had ended there in a difficult divorce. Still, as Mary once told me, "It was a wonderful time of my life. I was delighted with my art, and even more satisfied with my newfound role as mother."

But just as Mary's life seemed to be reaching a new stage, Brian called her with grim news: he'd tested positive for HIV, the virus that causes AIDS. He wanted Mary to know so she and Max, their then three-year-old son, could be tested, too. (Mary and Brian's other son, Zack, was adopted and not at risk.) It took Mary days to arrange to be tested. Afterward, she waited for the results. And waited. For two weeks, she waited to get her results—constantly calling the physician's office where she had been tested, always being told that "the results aren't available yet."

In late July, Mary was scheduled to join her parents, sisters, and brother for a family vacation. In a last-minute phone call from LaGuardia Airport she tried once more to reach the doctor who had tested her. When the nurse put the doctor on the line, Mary later reported, "I knew." Moments later, he confirmed what she feared: she had tested positive.

The daughter of Max Fisher, a well-known industrialist and philanthropist, she could have retreated into the comfortable wealth of her Detroit childhood. It could have been a secret shared with only her family and a handful of trusted friends. She could have been one of the nameless, faceless statistics chanted like some scientific mantra by "the experts." Mary could have denied that her body had been invaded by this most unwelcome visitor. She could have blocked it out and kept us all at a safe, comfortable distance.

But that's not Mary. If John Donne challenged, "Death be not proud"! Mary Fisher warns us all, "Life be not arrogant!" And she delivered her message in an unexpected forum. Who could forget the demure blonde at the podium of the 1992 Republican National Convention, speaking to a sea of delegates who moments earlier were smiling, waving signs, and whooping it up. Suddenly the only sound was Mary's voice, sweet yet strong. Her pain, so raw, her honesty, so riveting—a stark contrast to the dogmatic assertions that often characterize such gatherings. There was Mary, looking like a delicate angel, forcing everyone to hear what she had to say. Talking about AIDS in America—with the steely determination of the most ambitious politician present. Discussions of public policy and the economy, welfare reform and foreign affairs, all faded as everyone focused instead on just one woman who personified the hopes and dreams and anguish of so many.

No matter who you are, Mary Fisher is someone you'd like talking to. She's someone you'd be privileged to call your friend. I know I am. When you hear her voice on these pages, open your heart and your mind and realize there are countless Mary Fishers all around us; people who passionately want action, but, in the absence of that, would be grateful for the acknowledgment that AIDS exists and must be dealt with. People who desperately want research dollars, but will appreciate a simple hug. Mary Fisher—daughter, mother, AIDS activist, friend— deserves your attention. If you look carefully, you've probably already seen her. She is the woman browsing next to you in the bookstore. She's your son's high school French teacher. She's the policeman who's never told anyone he's gay, the poor woman in the "bad" part of town whose drug addiction has defeated her best intentions. She's the attorney who is losing weight, the bishop who has requested a transfer, the college senior who made a single, fatal mistake. She is the AIDS community. She is all of us. Mary makes it painfully clear that this is not a disease that happens to THEM. This is a disease that affects EVERYONE.

After paging through some of the speeches in this book, after crying, smiling, and praying for her, I remembered the Gospel according to Luke, which says we all have an obligation "through the tender mercy of our God, whereby the Dayspring from on high hath visited us, to give light to them that sit in darkness and in the shadow of death."

Every morning Mary wakes up in the shadow of death. She calls out her sons' names and holds them closely in her bed. From that moment on, she spends every hour seeking the strength and courage to fulfill her mission. Mary Fisher is a shining light for all of us who sit in darkness.

KATIE COURIC

I'LL NOT GO QUIETLY

LISTENING FOR ISAIAH

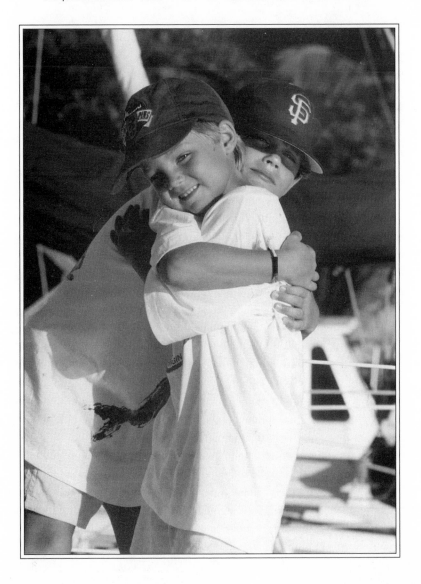

Brian Campbell Memorial Service
Provincetown Unitarian Church
Provincetown, Massachusetts
Saturday, September 25, 1993 (Yom Kippur)

––––––––

Brian died on Father's Day, June 20, 1993. Our relationship had healed in the months before his death. Sweet memories and the children had reclaimed stage center, nudging aside the bitterness that explains divorce.

After Brian's death, I needed a few months to resettle. The house in Florida had sold in June. The home to which the children and I were moving in Washington, D.C., wasn't ready until August. It was a thoroughly unsettled summer.

Then came September. Max headed off to conquer first grade and Zachary to master preschool. And I began shaping projects with Jim (A. James Heynen, the man who translates my ideas into plans and my passions into speeches).

I was grateful Brian's friends and family had asked me to speak at his memorial. It allowed me to name role models: Alice Foley, whose support had kept Brian hopeful during hard times; Manny Souza, Brian's nurse, who had wrapped medicine in gentle understanding; and Tina—Tina Campbell, Brian's sister— who had loved her brother, and the children, and me, through

the darkest hours. It was good to be in the church in Province-
town and remember Brian with those who'd loved him.

   And there was another, more distant audience I had in
mind. Someday Max and Zack may go looking for comfort.
They may wonder about Brian, or about me. In such mo-
ments, by leaving this record intact, I can encourage them—
at whatever age—to listen for Isaiah.

These are words from the prophet Isaiah:

> A voice says, "Cry!"
> And I said, "What shall I cry?"
> All flesh is grass,
> And all the beauty is like the flower of the field.
>
> The grass withers, the flower fades,
> When the breath of the Lord blows upon it;
> Surely the people is grass. . . .
>
> Comfort, comfort my people,
> Says your God.
> Speak tenderly to Jerusalem,
> And cry to her that her warfare is ended,
> That her iniquity is pardoned,
> That she has received from the Lord's hand
> Double gifts despite her sins. . . .
>
> Therefore . . .
> He will feed his flock like a shepherd,
> He will gather the lambs in his arms,
> He will carry them in his bosom,
> And gently lead those that are with young.

Comfort, comfort my people,
Says your God.
Speak tenderly to Jerusalem,
For her iniquity is pardoned.

Today is Yom Kippur. It is the day on which the chief high priest enters the Holy of Holies, the most sacred place in the temple, and there sprinkles uncontaminated blood on the ark of the covenant, offering a sacrifice to atone for the sins of God's people. Today is Yom Kippur, the Day of Atonement, the day our iniquity is pardoned and we celebrate the comfort of our forgiveness.

I did not know it would be Yom Kippur when we set aside this day for Brian's memorial. But I'm glad it is. And whether you are Jewish or Christian, religious or merely spiritual, it's a good day to remember that our comfort and our forgiveness are often wrapped tightly together.

We do not need a memorial service to remember. Every day, every night—sometimes, it seems, every hour—we remember the tilt of his head, the smoothness of his walk, his flashing smile or his sullen darkness, the humor that sizzled and the joke we didn't dare retell. Every day, it seems, new memories wash back, sometimes like a gentle and quiet rainfall, sometimes in a raging flood: some painful, some joyful, some that have been repressed and some that have been treasured. We don't need a service or a sanctuary to remember Brian.

But what we remember, and how; what feelings come along in the company of our memories, and what fears—these are worth a moment together in a place that reminds us of God.

We remember Brian's life and our relationships with him. We remember the morning when, half-dressed, he made his first, and last, attempt at putting a diaper on a giggling son—but he moved too slow, and the baby's aim was better than his; I remember that morning. We remember the sight of him racing across Boston Common when the boys were little, hiding behind the trees and inviting a chase; it was a golden, autumn day. We remember hard times and sharp words, soothing promises and long good-byes, quiet months and careful calls. We remember the closing days, the conversation we had always needed and nearly missed, the joy of hugging and the peace of forgiveness. We remember Brian's life.

Unless we live a life of mind-numbing denial, we also remember Brian's death: a father taken, a brother gone, a friend and husband no longer here. If by his life he brought us joy, and by his art he enriched our lives, then by his death he reminded us again of our own mortality. When we turn from his passing, we look in the mirror, and we know that he has only gone before us. For those who are HIV-positive, the mirror is brilliantly clear and, sometimes, terrifyingly close.

It's no wonder that we may want to skip quickly over the memories of pain and death. We blot out memories, hoping thereby to block out realities. But then, what's left is the tattered remnant of a relationship riddled with gaps and holes—without pain, perhaps, but also without truth or meaning.

If we are surviving only by avoidance, we would do better to reach out for atonement. It is God's recognition that the human condition is not easy, nor perfect, nor pain free. The flower fades, the grass withers, and surely all people are grass. A voice says, "Cry!" and I say, "What shall I cry?" And the next word we hear is . . . "comfort."

And if we focus too hard on the dying or too long on the AIDS or too frequently on those who pass easy judgment while we die hard—our lives become consumed by anger. For nearly every person with AIDS, there is someone they loved or trusted. There is terror enough to haunt our nights, stigma enough to fill our days, and anger enough—when it is swallowed—to poison our souls.

If we are wallowing in pools of anger, we would do better to remember Yom Kippur—to remember that our warfare is ended, that the word of forgiveness has been spoken, that the judgment of God is finally settled with a word of grace.

Most of us have learned the danger of avoidance; we've grown realistic—if only because there have been too many memorials. And most of us have found ways to resolve our anger, if only because it burned so hotly that it demanded resolution. What we have struggled with most, I think, is not avoidance, and not anger, but pure, grinding agony. We have been gripped by a terror so perfect—a sense that time is so fleeting, a grief that is so penetrating—that we are immobilized. We would welcome our own Day of Atonement, but we do not know how to achieve it. We cannot find a Holy of Holies, we have no healing high priest, there is no uncontaminated blood. And we are not quite sure where God has gone.

If I had a magic potion, a special comfort for the grieving—and if I had not used it all to heal the wounds in childish souls of two sons left behind—I would give it to you gladly. But I have none. What I have is only this conviction: if we cannot turn our faces away from death, then we must at least remember that death is not what God is really like.

God is more like the laughter that follows our sweeter memories, the quiet breeze that once lifted his favorite kite, the sunshine that filtered through the leaves above Brian's hiding place in Boston Common. God is more like the canvas that Brian started and the boys finished, in colors that they loved.

Or, if you would like to know what God is really like, consider Manny Souza and Alice Foley. In days of pain, their focus was comfort; in hours of distress and embarrassment, their only goals were peace and dignity. When Brian and I needed a night together, they were encouraging; and when we needed a stronger hand, they were there before we had asked. When Brian was uncertain, Manny was convincing; when all Tina or I could do was weep, Manny hugged us with quiet joy. When his struggle was over, and Brian was gone, it was Alice who brought comfort by opening a window. And it was Manny who lifted me from Brian and said, "Now that you know, you must tell them what it's like."

We would do well, as a company of pilgrims, to look toward the likes of Alice Foley and Manny Souza and whisper to God, "So this is what you are really like."

I suppose it will not be long before I hear the question, "Mommy, what was my daddy really like?"

I think that I will tell them about a kite that he once flew so high, it nearly kissed the sun. I think that I'll remember with them the sunrise hour when he held my hand steady and taught me how to use the brush. I may show them the picture I took of Brian running with them both—hoisted by the britches, one in each hand—until the three of them fell into a giggling heap. Or perhaps I'll take them to Boston Common and point across the green to the tree where, if they look quite closely, they may still catch a glimpse. And I may look around to you, his friends and family, with hope that you will take up the memories when I must put them down.

And if the day should come when they ask, "And what is God really like?" I may point them to the brightest star in the heavens, or a pair of earthbound caregivers who brought us grace. I will tell them about the Day of Atonement. And I will sit quietly with them, and listen, until together we hear Isaiah's voice again:

> He will feed his flock like a shepherd,
> He will gather the lambs in his arms,
> He will carry them in his bosom,
> And gently lead those that are with young.

WHEN IT MATTERS

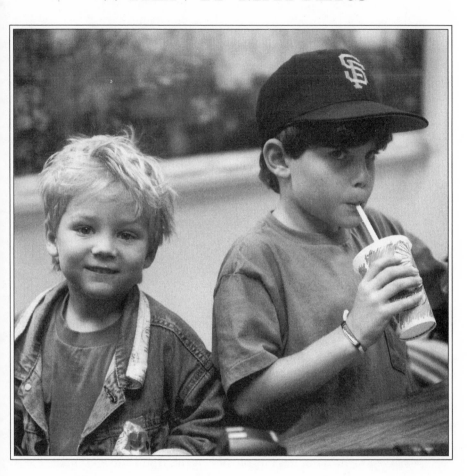

AIDS Caregivers
San Juan, Puerto Rico
Tuesday, September 28, 1993

———

The Puerto Rican Chamber of Commerce had organized an "AIDS in the Workplace" conference and invited me to speak. A few days later, an invitation to address a Special Session of the Puerto Rican Senate arrived (and was accepted). "And," we were told, "there'll be AIDS caregivers who want to meet with you."

I'd always wondered what it would be like to address a session of legislators. Now I know: it's great! My speech was broadcast throughout the legislative halls. When I stopped talking, senators started discussing what I'd said; when I left the hall, people stopped me to whisper encouragement.

The president of Puerto Rico's Senate had brought me into the chamber, as a means of raising AIDS awareness. What I had to say to his colleagues was specific: "The per capita rate of infections in Puerto Rico is higher than in any other territory in the States with the exception of Washington, D.C. . . . You are in a high-risk category, not a safety zone. Do not look away."

But what I had to say, later, to small groups of caregivers is what I've said to thousands like them in other places. If you're looking for a hero, find a caregiver in the nearest AIDS community. You won't have to look any farther.

The man whose AIDS virus I share is gone now. The memorial service was last week Saturday. We had been married, then divorced. We'd gone through long periods of silence and anger. And we had, in the final months, found our way to forgiveness.

"It's for the sake of the boys," we said at first, both to ourselves and to each other. For the children, we started speaking more frequently and more rationally. For the children, we needed to spend time together. But in the end, it was not for the children. It was for us. Though it was important for our children, Max and Zack, it mattered most to us—to Brian and Mary. We needed to find forgiveness.

The hardest thing for me to explain to many audiences—though surely not to this one—is that the AIDS virus does not fundamentally alter our lives or our characters. We struggle with our careers and our marriages, our divorces and our failings. Our children delight us and exhaust us. People with rotten, self-pitying personalities do not improve with AIDS, and folks with good humor and great grace usually retain their winning spirits. Broken families still need mending; tattered relationships still need attention; and the wounds we inflict on each other still heal only when wrapped in gentle forgiveness.

You and I know about the changes that accompany this disease: physical, emotional, economic, and spiritual. We know them too well because we see them every day. But for a moment I want to focus on what doesn't change.

What doesn't change is the need for acceptance, affection, and the sense that we matter. Being told that society cannot respect someone with this virus is hard; getting the message that the virus is God's judgment on us is harder. They are hard because of what has not changed: our need to feel accepted and loved and valued.

What doesn't change is the need for sustained relationships. In a constantly changing environment, especially when we are facing constantly changing needs, the permanence of some stable relationships is critical.

Our fear of dying doesn't change; neither does the delight in a glorious sunset or the taste of a child's kiss or the terror of being left alone or the smell of chocolate chip cookies in the oven or the agony of losing a loved one or the tears that come suddenly, without warning. The promise that comes with the first streak of morning sunlight can still revive our hopes, and an old friend's jokes on the telephone can still bring giggles.

What doesn't change, of course, is our need to be human. To have purpose. To feel the touch of someone's hand. To know that, if we were gone, someone would notice and care. To imagine that we might have made a difference. To believe that someone will remember us.

And here's where you all come in. You care for those who grow weary of needing care, and you keep caring. You listen to us when we repeat ourselves, endlessly. You help us find dignity, when others are trying to hide it from us—and we seem intent on throwing it away ourselves. You keep us focused on life, when death is erasing all the familiar names from our address books.

I'll tell you a story. The same day her favorite grandson began kindergarten, a grandmother—fighting the ravages of cancer—moved into a nursing home. And so, to raise her spirits, her grandson began making her a gift in school. With every ounce of dexterity five-year-old fingers could muster, he assembled a delicate masterpiece from toothpicks and tiny crystal figurines.

When last week Friday his parents came to visit his classroom, the kindergartener couldn't restrain himself. He went dashing through the crowd of children and, just short of his parents, he tripped and fell and grandma's gift was shattered into a thousand hapless pieces.

His father, loving him deeply and sensing his enormous hurt, bent down and whispered, "It doesn't matter, Son; Grandma knows you love her." But his mother, in a moment of wiser grace, picked him up and cried with him. "I know," she said, "I know . . . it matters. It matters very much."

I thank you for all the unseen and uncounted ways in which you've told and shown members of the AIDS community you know that they matter.

And, beyond my thanks, comes this quiet prayer: When next you are on the emotional edge, ready to give up, practicing your speech on "burnout"—may you hear God's voice calling, "I know you're weary. But don't go, because you matter. You matter very much."

If you hear a second voice, it might be mine, saying, "Don't leave me without a hug." Thanks for letting me be a part of your day.

THE
LOOKING-GLASS COMMUNITY

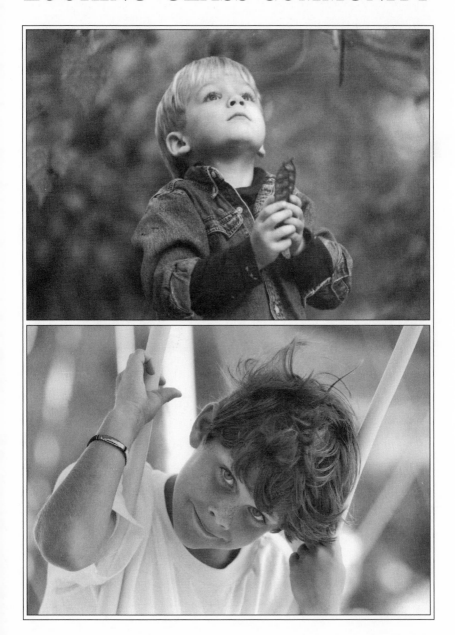

1993 National Hospice Organization
Annual Symposium and Exposition
Opening Address
Salt Lake City, Utah
Friday, October 15, 1993

———

Every speech tackles death, because every speech is composed inside the AIDS community where death hangs out on every corner.

Where death is, hospices have sprung up in recent years. They've provided homes of hope during a time of hopelessness. They've taught us much about living by helping us reckon with our dying. They're staffed with extraordinary people like Pat Gibbons, whom I'd met when I was on the National Commission on AIDS and who, later, introduced me to the meaning of hospice during Brian's illness.

In the weeks before this speech, ABC's Nightline *with Ted Koppel had moved into our family's life for an extended period. The speech let me recall that event with some joy.*

It also let me, for the first time, try saying in public what had happened to me when I went to death's doorstep with

Brian. Like every AIDS caregiver who is also AIDS infected, I
had found myself looking squarely into a mirror.

Hospice the organization, hospice the movement, and hospice the idea—all have played such positive roles in the life of
our society that I imagine you've gathered with a sense of enormous pride. At least, I hope you have. If I had only one minute
to address you and one thing to tell you, I'd tell each of you to
go to a quiet place and sit for an hour in silent reflection on all
that you've accomplished. Before you take up your theme, "The
challenges of change," you could spend an hour recognizing the
challenges you've met and the changes you've already
achieved. You are, together, an extraordinary group. I salute
each of you for the role you play in your critical campaign, and
I thank you for letting me share these moments with you.

Salt Lake City is my first public venue since being the subject of an ABC *Nightline* special a few Friday evenings ago. For
three weeks, a production crew had moved into my life—and I
mean, moved in *everywhere:* from public auditoriums and private telephone conversations to the intimacy of my studio and
the quiet of my children's bedrooms. Some people suppose
there's a sense of honor in all this. Perhaps there is. Mainly, for
me, there's a sense of mission—mission, and terrifying vulner-
ability.

I've spent my years as a television producer. I know what
cameras and microphones can capture and portray. For the
sake of getting out the message, having a crew move in with us
was certainly worthwhile. But knowing that ten or twenty million people were going to have a peek into our family's most intimate moments certainly gave me a moment or two of hard
thought.

I mean . . . *you* may be a beauty queen or quarterback candidate when you wake up in the morning; but walking out of my bedroom in a rumpled bathrobe after a sleepless night with two children with the flu, desperate for coffee, remembering that cameras are waiting for me, I didn't feel especially stunning that morning.

And if *my* patience wore thin, I was absolutely a hero by comparison to my two sons. Do you know that a four-year-old boy really doesn't care about Ted Koppel's ratings when he wants five minutes alone with his mother? And a six-year-old, given an audience of five adults with cameras and sound equipment, might just decide to try out "those words" that his older friend taught him? Did someone say this was all "an *honor*"? I'm not so sure.

David Kennerly, a dear friend and a Pulitzer Prize–winning photojournalist, had originally conceived the project. He knew how strongly I believe in communicating the realities of HIV and AIDS, and he knew that I trusted him to do it. And if there is any praise to be distributed for that program, David has earned the lion's share.

My affection for David was enhanced not only by what *was* aired, but also by what was *not*. During the third week of our experiment with communal living, Kennerly decided the weather was perfect for some shots of my sons playing with me outside in the yard. So there—in full view of a Pulitzer Prize winner, an ABC camera crew, Ted Koppel's producer, and God—the boys got into the ugliest little brawl you've ever imagined. In a scene reminiscent of all great American families, Zack wanted to kill Max, and Max started using "those words" again. I responded as any good mother would under these conditions: I ranted and raved, hollered and screamed, and did everything Dr. Spock assured us would transform our children into felons—and I did this with a microphone clipped to my blouse, in living color, for the world to see.

I was remembering these moments of glory those few Friday evenings ago, waiting for *Nightline* to come on the air. I was somewhere between palpable anxiety and numbing terror, prepared to have my very worst private moments exposed on national television. What I was not prepared for, I think, was the more vulnerable emotion that actually swept over me as I watched.

The program opened at Brian's grave. The man I'd known as a husband—my children's father, the person whose virus I shared—had died on Father's Day. The ABC crew was with us when the boys and I went back to visit his grave for the first time, and they opened the *Nightline* show with those scenes. All the zaniness of the three weeks disappeared, and I was transported back in time.

There I was kneeling with Max and Zack, pushing aside dirt on Brian's grave, holding little hands and missing a larger one.

And then, there I was, sitting in my breakfast room, starting to cry while trying to explain how hard it is to answer my children's questions about my own life, and my own AIDS.

And then, there I was, at Brian's memorial service, remembering the words of the prophet Isaiah: "'What shall I cry?' And the voice said, 'Comfort.'"

What's important for you to hear this morning is not only that I was there, but I was not there alone. Do you know who else was there? You were.

You were there in the person of Pat Gibbons, whose wisdom and strength had helped me prepare for the impossible and to be strong during the unendurable. You were there when I arrived at Brian's apartment in those last days, in the caregiver who quietly explained to me the signs of death, giving me an understanding I did not want but could not serve without. You were there in the young man who quietly watched over us, when Brian's hands—his graceful, artist's hands; the hands with which he'd shown me how to hold a brush and into which I'd placed a firstborn son—you were there when his hands began to stiffen. And you were there, in the stronger hands of the caregiver who lifted me from his bed long after the breathing had stopped.

I am here today, above all else, to say thank you; to tell you that you were there in my life at a time and place where no one else could have done what you did. You did much more than bring dignity to death; you helped bring meaning to life. And I am also here today to say your work is not yet finished, not in my life and not in the life of our nation. In some senses, it may have just begun.

You have gathered in the shadow of the everlasting hills to consider "the challenges of change." And you are an example of this change: *hospice* was itself an unknown term not long ago, certainly within most of our lifetimes. And think of AIDS, a disease just being named a decade ago that has already achieved its status as the most deadly epidemic in human history. We live in a time of unstoppable change.

In such a context, you will grow. As more and more of us reach out toward hospice, more and more of you will need to respond. Finances must be generated and people must be equipped. In the course of this seemingly endless mission, there are those among you who may grow weary. You have been on the front lines since the first shot was fired. You've explained the meaning of hospice not only in brochures, but in actions; you have moved from bedrooms to boardrooms, demonstrating that your mission is focused on living not dying. You have worn yourselves down in the effort to build up our spirits.

A year ago I, with a few friends and one extraordinary brother, established an organization known as the Family AIDS Network. Most of our work in the past year has been aimed at building AIDS awareness within communities—local, regional, and national. But in the coming months, one of our planned goals will be realized when we implement the Caregiver Award program, an award for which many of you are eligible. We will ask the National Hospice Organization to join with other partners in identifying those caregivers who have done heroic things in the name of ordinary service. We will seek out those who have devoted their lives to caring for others and place them on the stage of national attention—not merely for the sake of notoriety or fame, but for the purpose of consciousness-raising. The nation needs to know that many of our heroes are to be found not on the battlefield nor on the athletic field, but in the field of healing and affection. The hospice worker who brings comfort and peace, the caregiver who wipes tears and cleans the laundry, the gentle provider who carries us through nights of immeasurable agony while we live out the final days with someone we love—these are heroes worthy of admiration and emulation.

Community is a fragile creature. We have broken it with our emphasis on race and class, creed and gender. We have taught our children to fear those who are unlike us in the pigment of their skin or the content of their wallet. We have drawn red lines on white real estate maps to keep black neighbors from moving in. Even in our dying, we have maintained our well-defined patterns of segregation and discrimination, from the social services that ease our suffering to the funeral home that retrieves the body.

We threaten a community's life when, with great ease, we begin dividing between "we" and "they"—as if we are choosing sides for a softball game. When there is a "we," and "we" are only responsible for ourselves, community has gone from being fragile to being fractured. When all sense of personal responsibility ends at the edge of our property lines or the bottom of our checkbook balances; when AIDS is seen as a disease of "those people," of people who are "like that"—tell me, what has become of community?

Community is woven from the threads of human life. And the worth of a human life is itself, sometimes, quite fragile. Those who pay taxes are regarded as contributors; they are good—implying that any who cannot pay, who may be "cash drains" in our society, are evil. Those who are strong in ability and body, who go to work in the morning and to their children's schools in the evening—these are our preferred neighbors and friends—Is it because we've judged them more worthy than those who bear a mental illness or have lost their employment?

It can be frightening to contemplate how, precisely, we appear to measure human worth. In a culture that venerates beauty and strength and athletic grace, that admires the flashing smile and the tanned good looks of youth—the worth of a homeless, dying man is not altogether certain. In a culture where more cash is devoted in one month to cosmetic surgery, fad diets, and teenage liposuction than will be spent in an entire year on AIDS research—the worth of a single mother with two children and one virus is, I suppose, not altogether certain.

Community is a fragile creature, and we are called to nurture it, to help it grow vigorously and grow strong.

Human worth is an immeasurable commodity, and we are called to invest in it, to give it not only dignity but meaning.

To help strengthen community and nurture human worth I would like to offer three requests on behalf of those who, like me, are HIV-positive: the pilgrims on the road to AIDS.

My first request is that, in your important work with hospice, you do all you can to have the realities of your service match the ideals of your promise. I know your formal position is one of acceptance and care for those with AIDS, and I also know that it has sometimes been hard to achieve the full intent of this promise.

I speak as a friend and admirer, and as an adult: we all seek standards in our lives that are sometimes hard to achieve; we all know the taste of some failure and disappointment. But, because I represent a pilgrim band that struggles enough, I urge you to do what you can to translate the promise of care into the reality of treatment for those who suffer AIDS in your communities.

At one extreme, there are those who have less fear of death than of homosexuality. Many dying today come from the gay community. Seeing them in our midst, we can feel how fragile a creature community really is; seeing one member of the gay community wasting and dying, we must answer our own questions of human worth. But if fear of those who are gay has become a shadow over a hospice program, preventing it from fully flowering in comfort and joy for those who are most in need—I urge you, break down the walls of discrimination and fear. Do it because you love community, because human beings have worth, and because we live the most satisfied when we live with most integrity.

At the other extreme are those who think working with the AIDS community has a certain celebrity attached to it. We leave our gleaming kitchens and comfortable homes and, Mother Teresa-like, become the ministers to those who are outcasts in society. It's the sort of thing we like to mention, casually, while sipping Evian at a cocktail party on the way to the theatre. But it's not the motivation that will hold during hours that are hard.

On behalf of millions of pilgrims on the road to AIDS, I urge you to open the doors of hospice not only to the *promise* of care for those with AIDS, but to the *reality*. If it would help to have HIV-positive people on your staff, contact a local AIDS organization. If it would help to run training services or educational programs, ask for assistance. But, please, don't let the promise go unfulfilled in your community.

My second request is simply that you see those who are my fellow pilgrims on the road to AIDS for what we are: a looking-glass community. We are the people who, when someone dies of AIDS, see ourselves and our future. You might have peeked through a window into Brian's bedroom during those final hours, but I was peering into a looking-glass, bearing not only the grief of his final hours but a recognition about my own. In seeing where they must walk, all of us who are HIV-positive see where we will follow. When their blood counts grow less happy, we think of our own. When yesterday's breakfast companion is struck with pneumonia during the night, we clear our throats uncomfortably. When Sunday's party is over, and on Monday we go to the bedside of a gifted writer whose brain is now clouded by infection, whose eyes are eager yet sad, we wonder where the virus will finally strike us; how—exactly *how*—will it hit me?

When I hear the slurs against those who are gay or the judgments passed on those who used drugs, I feel the sting of discrimination—living in a looking-glass community, I cannot see them without seeing myself reflected. We cannot walk through this crowd judging between the guilty and the innocent, the worthwhile and the worthless. If you reject my gay brothers or my weakened sisters, you reject me. Because I live in a looking-glass community.

When Charles Williams died, C. S. Lewis—for whom Williams was a most special friend—wrote a stunning poem, which samples the agony that today hangs over the AIDS community. Lewis's poem could easily have described the aching void left, say, by the loss of Arthur Ashe:

> Your death blows a strange bugle call,
> friend, and all is hard
> To see plainly or record truly. The new
> light imposes change,
> Readjusts all a life-landscape as it thrusts
> down its probe from the sky,
> To create shadows, to reveal waters, to
> erect hills and deepen glens.
> The slant alters. I can't see the old
> contours. . . .
>
> Is it the first sting of the great winter, the
> world-waning? Or the cold of spring?
> A hard question and worth talking a
> whole night on. But with whom?
> Of whom now can I ask guidance? With
> what friend concerning your death
> Is it worth while to exchange thoughts
> unless—oh, unless it were you?

When you are serving my fellow pilgrims, remember that those of us who love the dying are often, ourselves, only a small measure behind them. And we come to you, hospice, hoping for your comfort.

And my third request is simple. I would like you to serve not only those of us who are pilgrims on the road to AIDS, but also our children. My own sons are perfectly ordinary: they are my delight and joy, and my terror in the night, bright, independent, too outspoken in one moment and far too quiet in the next. Neither is HIV-positive. Both are on course to become orphans.

And nothing is likely to alter that course early enough to make the critical difference.

When you, the community of comfort, embrace us, the looking-glass community, you may notice a host of children. They are too young to be like you—strong, wise, and capable of understanding the meaning of life and the challenge of death. They will understand something of pain and suffering, but little of hope and healing. And they will not be old enough when the time comes.

If we do not wait until the hour of death to challenge the ugly stereotypes of persons with AIDS, that will make it easier. If you would return to your communities to oppose those who regard AIDS as a death sentence earned by behavior, I would be grateful. Do it now, before the fragile communities are shattered and human worth must be dug out of the debris.

And if, in the days ahead, I should be one of the pilgrims who grows weary and needs to rest, then I will come back to you again, hospice. I will come that day not to say thank you, but to say please. I will come with a child in each hand, preparing to place their hands into yours. I will do it with hope, because I have seen the strength of your comfort in the months that have just gone by. And I will do it with courage, because you have helped me learn that it is life that yields our dignity, not death.

And when that hour has passed, I will be grateful to know that it is you who will answer Max's question, "Why?" and that it is you to whom Zack can turn when asking where his mother has gone. In their grief and your grace, they will hear an echo of C. S. Lewis.

Of whom else could they ask guidance? With what friend concerning my death "is it worth while to exchange thoughts / unless—oh, unless it were you?"

Now, for the hours of your conference and the days of your service: grace to you, and peace.

SEW ME A MEMORY

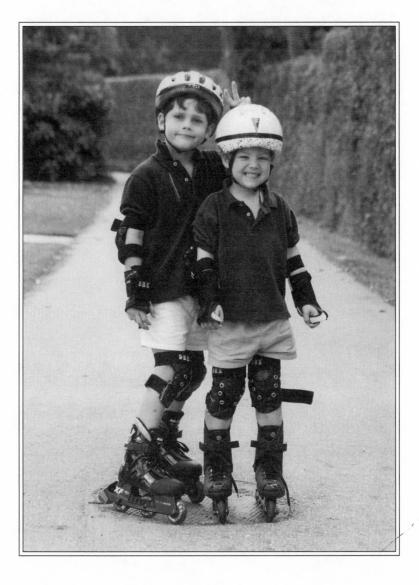

Opening Ceremonies for
the NAMES Project AIDS Memorial Quilt
Jewish Community Center
Houston, Texas
Sunday, October 17, 1993

———

*The AIDS national monument, the Quilt, was at the Jewish
Community Center in Houston to accompany an AIDS awareness week. It had been more than a year since I'd spoken at the
Republican National Convention in this city—and since the
moment a strapping young man had peeled off his long-
sleeved shirt to show the world a T-shirt reading, "No one here
knows I'm HIV-positive." His name: Steven Bradley.*

*Now, a year later, Steven Bradley had helped arrange the
Quilt's appearance and mine. I was honored to be invited. Be-
sides, going to Houston meant spending hours with Steven—
zany hours full of hearty laughter and big meals and great
affection, touching the fabric of the Quilt and weaving together the fabric of our lives.*

*Steven Bradley is dead now. I took the news hard, when it
came. Some friends sent a copy of his memorial in a packet,
and I wouldn't open it—I didn't want his death confirmed in
writing.*

In a tangle of children and questions and confusion, the
packet was ripped open one afternoon a few weeks after it had
arrived. Contents spilled across my bedroom floor. I turned
over a stray piece of white fabric, and my breathing stopped. It
was Steven's T-shirt. "No one here knows . . ."

I held it as I would have held Steven. And I wept as I had
not wept since Brian died.

We've gathered today at the national memorial for those who
have fallen in the battle with AIDS. Some were small and
young, born to a life haunted by blood tests and hospitals from
beginning to end. Some were children or young people, never
knowing quite how they came to be where they were. Some were
celebrities; most were not. Some were famous; most never knew
the public limelight. They were, by and large, like us: ordinary
people who suffered what is becoming a most ordinary illness,
stolen from life during the prime of their lives and ours. They
were our teachers and our mates, our colleagues and our
friends, our brothers and sisters—they were, to say it most simply, people we loved.

Remembering those who are memorialized in the panels of
the Quilt is something done in the spirit of our nation. To visit
the Quilt is, after all, to visit a national memorial. Although
they have fallen in a battle, those whose names are posted here
did not enlist; all were drafted, reluctantly, into a war not of
their making, thrust on them against their will. They were
drawn from every race and color, every community and context.
They were armed by conscience and by companionship, but
they were not armed by their nation, nor has their nation decorated them for any service they performed.

And so we have come to a national memorial, as haunting

as—and with numbers far greater than—Washington's long wall inscribed with the names of those who died in Vietnam. The long black wall is, indeed, a wall of mourning; but if there is any hope to be found in it, it is this: we do not add names to the Vietnam memorial each morning. But the Quilt continues to grow by the day and, to be more precise, by the hour.

Until the Quilt is finished, it is wise for those of us who remain to gather at the memorial from time to time, if only to remember—not so much for those who have fallen as for ourselves. Those who have gone before us no longer need our memories; it is we who need the recollections, we who must draw the lessons from history that have not yet been learned.

And so, as we walk quietly among the panels, we must remember the voice that has been silenced. As we experience the community of grief, seen in the hugs we exchange and the tears we shed while pausing among the panels, we must remember that we are bound together with bands of love that cannot be broken.

For many of us, it is not possible to stroll casually onto the floor that holds the Quilt. No matter how often we have been in its presence, we come to the Quilt tentatively, reverently, as one comes into the presence of something greater than oneself. We move from panel to panel, not only remembering but wondering. We see a name and we ask, "Why?" An image triggers a flood of memories, and we wonder, "Is there any purpose in all this? Is it simply, merely, mindless suffering?" Like the blanket tossed by a restless sleeper, the Quilt can raise hard questions for those who are willing to wonder.

Some of those who come to the Quilt have already faced the harder question. We are HIV-positive and we have wanted an answer to the simple question "Why me?" We have shaken our fists and screamed it; we have gone to our knees and begged it. I do not think it is possible to be HIV-positive, and reasonable, and not wonder about the answer. "Why us?" asks the parent whose child needed the lifesaving transfusion; in choosing for her daughter's life, has a mother earned a slower sentence to death? The man who never knew there was a terminal risk in a loving relationship and the woman who trusted her husband—no matter how or where or why the infection found us, the question that arrived not long after was the same: "Why, and why me?"

As it happened, I learned I was HIV-positive during a time of my life in which I was especially spiritually sensitive. Perhaps that's why, from the beginning, I've believed that all things in life are given for a purpose. But even so, it is no easy belief. My confidence that there is *some* purpose has not reduced the urgency with which I ask, "What might that purpose be?"

If I am unsure what the purpose *is,* I am certain what the purpose is *not:* it is not God's judgment. Lung cancer is not caused by sin and damnation, even when the cancer patient smoked cigarettes. I do not believe God sits in heaven, spotting smokers and "getting them." I do not imagine that men who eat large steaks with heavy loads of salt are earning God's wrath, which spins them into a heart attack. And I do not think God spent eternity devising AIDS as a peculiar form of suffering for a few of his children. In truth, I believe quite the opposite. I believe God cares for those who suffer, even if their own weaknesses helped contribute to the suffering. If there is special condemnation, it is reserved for those who are self-righteous, who trade in hatred and engage in the abuse of others. Therefore, I believe, the names inscribed on the Quilt belong to God's children, not to objects of God's wrath.

Perhaps, I've sometimes thought, the purpose of all this suffering will be found in our response to it. Perhaps AIDS will be the instrument by which we will learn, as a nation if not as a world, that we are interdependent and interrelated. "Maybe," I've said to myself, "the fact that all of us are at risk for this illness will teach us something of our commonality." If that were true, then, seeing our own frailty, we will be less ready to judge the weakness of another. And if that were true, then—when the one and a half or two million Americans now HIV-positive grow sick and die—perhaps then, I've thought, the conscience of the nation will come to life. This is, in general, my most optimistic view.

The difficulty with this view, of course, is how little evidence we have to support it. After more than a decade of life in the midst of this epidemic, instead of recognizing our interdependence and our interrelatedness, the belief persists that AIDS is a disease of "those people," not "us."

What hopeful evidence is there that the growth of this epidemic is fostering growth of brotherhood and compassion? In the face of staggering suffering with infections reported in unprecedented numbers and spreading at astounding rates, communities have refused educational programs that would save the lives of their children. Little ones with AIDS have been denied admission to schools. Parents with AIDS have been removed from employment, their only source of health care and insurance. People of all ages have been denied access to every human service from simple dental care to the final attention of the local undertaker. And the gay community, already the object of profound abuse, has been given another reason to fear battering.

There is some evidence that *fear* of dying has moved some people to take precautions, and that shame has terrorized a few others. And we can see that, once we saw AIDS leaving the gay community, America's majority population took a much livelier interest in risk factors.

But let us, in the shadow of the national memorial to AIDS,

be truthful. Unnecessary shame and raw self-interest do not equal compassion, and fear of dying is no evidence of a sensitive conscience. If AIDS is to be an instrument of human understanding, we have not yet begun to see its purpose fulfilled.

I have no simple answer to the question "Why me?" And, in the end, I do not know where to find meaning within the AIDS epidemic. I am not sure, for all that I have thought about it, that I understand it well at all.

But I understand this: Until we have stirred the nation's conscience, we will not have the weapons with which to wage a successful battle against AIDS. Until we have captured the soul of the nation, we will not have its commitment to press for a cure, demand a preventative, and call for compassion in the place of stigma and discrimination. It is important to call for sound legislation, but it is not enough. It is mandatory to press for decent care through channels of law and justice, but it will not be enough. Until justice rolls down from the walls of the temple, and righteousness flows from the doors of the churches, we are not yet defeating the spiritual cause which flowers in indifference and insensitivity, that gives root to stigma and refuge to discrimination, that justifies our prejudices and decorates our ignorance. We must find ways to stir the nation's conscience by touching souls.

And in this effort, the Quilt has a special role to play. As a living memorial, tragically growing on an hourly basis, the Quilt gives mounting evidence of the toll taken by this epidemic. Dancers who no longer leap and turn; writers whose pens have dropped from listless hands; children whose gifts were squandered; brothers and sisters whose love was taken from us—all are remembered in the names nestled into panels of the Quilt.

As its sections go from city to city, this memorial reminds us that our future is being put at risk by a clear and present danger today. It calls for moral courage on the part of those who create curricula and raise children, for integrity on the part of those who mount pulpits and preach hope, and for leadership on the part of those who set our communities' agenda and report the communities' news.

The Quilt plays a critical role in the nation's education. But there is more that it can do, because the panels stretched from corner to corner serve not only as a lesson in our ongoing history; they also issue a muted plea for understanding.

The Quilt may not, itself, produce a cure; but it can ask that we live with compassion. In hearing the names and seeing the panel, a distant voice may call to those who've never heard before. And if the voice is true, and they are ready to hear, they will know that those who died were no strangers in this land: They were the kid sister who joked at the family table, the uncle who brought the special holiday cheer, the child whose grin could make us all smile, the one we loved—whose voice we still hear in our dreams. To be enshrined on a panel of the Quilt is no peculiar honor, nor is it any shame; it is merely to be remembered—no more, and no less. When the names are being read, the Quilt is given a voice. And those who hear it, will hear the call to compassion.

For those who share my virus—all those who are HIV-positive— the Quilt has a special poignancy. In remembering those who have gone before us, we see that every life has purpose and value, including our own. In hearing the names of those who have died, we remember that the meaning and legacy attached to our names will come in our living, not in our dying. As we walk amid the panels and our memories, we remember that we are human, no more and no less. And we remember this: that we are called to live with hope—not because we have all the answers, but because we have faith. And faith is the ability to live hopefully *without* the answers.

And so I invite you all to join me at this national memorial. To those of you who, like me, are pilgrims on the road to AIDS, I extend a special invitation to reach out. Reach out to touch the Quilt, knowing that it is a memorial also to our spirit and to our courage. See the Quilt as a banner of hope, not a shroud of shame. Take hold of its promise and be lifted up in its beauty.

And do not run from us, even when you have reached for the Quilt; reach also for us. If you dare not say it out loud, whisper your name to us. Embrace us with grief or joy, but do not leave this place until you have held us tightly, both for the strength you will receive and for the comfort you will give. Do not walk too quietly among us, lest each of us who is HIV-positive begin to believe that he or she is alone.

To those of you who are caregivers, who have cared for those who've gone before us and care for us still, I offer a word of hope and courage. You grow weary of caring for those who are needy, and we grow weary of needing care; but we must not let weariness tear down our resolve or erode our strength. We must not burn out, because the battle has hardly begun. We cannot go on alone; we must have each other. We must infuse each other with new hope and find, between us, the courage to go on.

Therefore, take hold of the Quilt as a blanket of comfort with which to be warmed while you rest. Reach not only for the memories of pain and death, but—beyond them—to the enduring smile and the promise that you made . . . to remember. And, having remembered, leave your pain here. Do not walk from the Quilt carrying the agony of loss for those whose love you kindled and now miss. In the quiet passageways between the silent panels, do not fear the rage that fills your soul until it feels as if

it may burst; lay it down. Let it go. Give it up. In the security of
this community, the company of the committed, let go of that
which threatens to consume you. By giving up the anger and the
pain, you may make of the Quilt not only a memorial to those
who have fallen but also a relief for those who are left. Then we
may go out, again, to serve, refreshed.

For those who've come to demonstrate concern and love; for
leaders of our communities and clergy in our religious traditions; for those who seek compassion for the fallen and dignity
for the defamed—for those who are here as an act of solidarity
with those who are no longer here—I ask for your attention.
Look around you, not only at the Quilt but at the quiltmakers. If
you cannot promise them a cure, give them your conscience, so
that—when, together, we walk away from the Quilt—we will
promise each other decency and concern in the place of discrimination and misunderstanding.

And to those who have come only to grieve—to remember
his name and say it aloud once again, to hear her voice mur-
muring in your soul; to visit memories stitched into your heart
in patterns no Quilt can capture; to feel again the love that grew
so painful in the darkest hours—I invite you to do what you've
come to do: grieve. Grieve without fear and without shame.
Grieve without holding in or holding back. Grieve with those
who are near you, grieve with those who cannot stand at all.
Grieve, and remember that there is nothing that needs to divide
us from those we love—neither in life nor in death.

And should the hour come that I am no longer able to visit,
and that those who grieve include my children, I have a simple
request to make of you: help them to sew me a memory. Tell
them that I was human, no more and no less. Tell them that
once I came to issue a call not for pity, but for compassion.
Steady their hands as they draw a picture or write a poem. Offer

them a scrap of cloth and a needle and a touch of your courage
. . . so they can sew me a memory for their healing.

Until then, we can go to the Quilt together, you and I. There
we can remember that those who have fallen are not merely
numbered; they are named.

Let us go to the Quilt together, knowing that we have no
stronger hope for tomorrow than the commitment we have made
today.

Let us go to the Quilt together, to walk among our memories,
weep among the panels, and pray that one of us will still be
here when the last panel is being sewn into this grim and glorious national memorial.

Until that day, grace to you, and peace.

To
WORSHIP IN THE ASHES

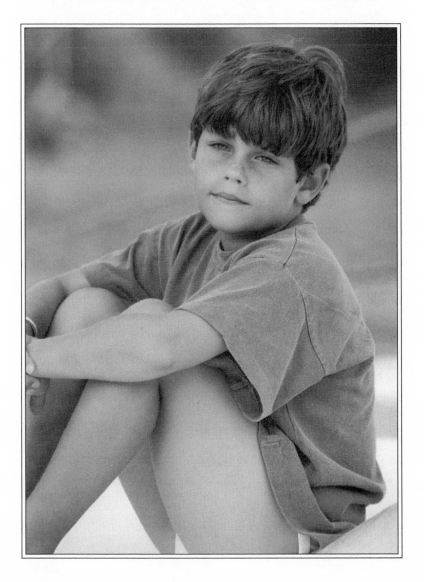

———

I first preached this sermon on September 12, 1993, at Rev. Christopher Hamlin's Sixteenth Street Baptist Church in Birmingham, Alabama, on the thirtieth anniversary of the bombing of that church by Ku Klux Klansmen. Families of Sunday-school children who'd been killed were present. "What can I say of forgiveness to the Sixteenth Street Baptist Church?" I asked them. "White men oppressed you as white women cheered them on. Under cover of darkness, white cowards planted the bomb that took your children's lives. And on the day you've set aside to remember, you invite me—a white woman—to stand before you, not to be judged but to worship with you."

When the First AME Church of Los Angeles invited me to preach a few months later, I didn't anticipate that the second preaching would be even more dramatic than the first.

I was tentative when I arrived at First AME, but Rev. Cecil "Chip" Murray soon made me welcome. Before I mounted the pulpit, the Reverend Mr. Murray and his colleagues laid their hands on me and prayed that I would speak God's word. Throughout the sermon, the congregation before me and the robed

*brothers and sisters behind me shouted encouragement.
"Preach it, Sister." "Say it out." "Tell them the truth now." It
was a chorus in which I spoke a line and they sang out responses.*

*Midway through my sermon, the organist softly played "We
Shall Overcome." As the volume came up and the congregation came to its feet, clapping and swaying, I began to regret
that it was over. When everyone sat down again and I heard a
voice behind me call out, "Preach it, Sister," I was elated.
Nothing had ended—we'd just paused for a brief celebration.*

*At the close of the service the men and women in robes bent
over me again in prayer, this time in a service of healing. And
what I felt, as I've never felt it before, was the power of their
prayer and the touch of their hands and the presence of God.*

SCRIPTURE READING

There was a man in the land of Uz, whose name was Job; and
that man was blameless and upright, one who feared God, and
turned away from evil. . . . this man was the greatest of all the
people of the east.

. . . the Lord said to Satan, "Have you considered my servant
Job, that there is none like him on the earth, a blameless and
upright man, who fears God and turns away from evil?" Then
Satan answered the Lord, ". . . Thou hast blessed the work of
his hands and his possessions have increased in the land. But
[take away] all that he has, and he will curse thee to thy face."

. . . Now there was a day when his sons and daughters were
eating and drinking wine in their eldest brother's house; and
there came a messenger to Job and said, "The oxen were plowing and the asses feeding beside them; and the Sabéans fell
upon them and took them, and slew the servants with the edge
of the sword; and I alone have escaped to tell you."

While he was yet speaking, there came another, and said, "The fire of God fell from heaven and burned up the sheep and the servants, and consumed them; and I alone have escaped to tell you."

While he was yet speaking, there came another, and said, "The Chaldéans formed three companies, and made a raid upon the camels and took them, and slew the servants with the edge of the sword; and I alone have escaped to tell you."

While he was yet speaking, there came another, and said, "Your sons and daughters were eating and drinking wine in their eldest brother's house; and behold, a great wind came across the wilderness, and struck the four corners of the house, and it fell upon the young people, and they are all dead; and I alone have escaped to tell you."

Then Job arose, and rent his robe, and shaved his head, and fell upon the ground, and worshiped. And he said, "Naked I came from my mother's womb, and naked shall I return; the Lord gave, and the Lord has taken away; blessed be the name of the Lord."

In all this Job did not sin or charge God with wrong.

[The Book of Job 1:1, 3, 8–11, 13–22]

The story of Job is well known in both of our traditions.

He was a man of great wealth and great reputation, "the greatest of all the people" of his community—a father who loved his children, a believer who loved his God. So honorable was Job, so strong and decent, that God bragged about him in a conversation with Satan.

"No wonder he's so fond of you," said the devil; "you've given him everything he could want. But take away all that he has and he'll curse you to your face."

"Not true," said God. And then came the awful proof.

The animals that would have plowed his fields and pulled the reapers were stolen; he could no longer farm. The sheep that would have clothed his family with wool and fed them in the wintertime were killed by lightning; he would be cold and hungry. The camels he could have traded, or on which he could have traveled to a new place, were lost in a raid. And after losing all his possessions, all his wealth, and all his capacity to gain them back, he suffered the worst loss: his children. "They are all dead," said the lone surviving servant—"They are all dead."

In the awful silence that follows such news, Job staggered to his feet. He took his robe in his hands and tore it from his breast. He cut the hair from his head so that, in the desert heat, he'd have nothing to shade himself, no place to hide. And—just when we're ready to read that he fell upon his sword and died— we read instead: "And he fell upon the ground . . . and worshiped."

"Naked I came from my mother's womb, and naked shall I return; the Lord gave, and the Lord has taken away; blessed be the name of the Lord."

The Book of Job looms over my Jewish and your Christian tradition like a great question mark: What do we say—and what do we do—when the innocent suffer? Though the story is ancient, the question is painfully modern. We cannot read recent history through the eyes of a Jewish child without smelling the smoke of Auschwitz and Dachau, without asking ourselves: What do we say? We cannot read the history of America through the eyes of an African-American child without smelling the smoke of a burning cross, or hearing the rattle of slavery's chains, and asking ourselves: What do we say?

Job's wife had a suggestion: "Curse God and die." What we don't know is the tone of voice in which she spoke.

If we think of her as a mean woman, we hear her getting rid

of a husband who's lost everything he offered her; but it isn't meanness that tempts us most to curse God and die.

If we think of her as a reasonable woman, we hear her giving common sense: "Just end it, Job. You're sick and poor and may as well stop suffering." But it isn't reason that tempts us most to curse God and die.

But suppose she comes only as a loving wife. Suppose her voice is full of compassion and grief. Suppose she goes to him—sitting in the ashes, scratching his open sores, naked—gently lifts his face in her hands and says, "Oh, Honey . . . curse God, so you can die." When the innocents suffer, those who love them may suffer more. It is love that makes us most vulnerable to pain.

In the hillsides and canyons surrounding this sanctuary, the searing heat and acid smoke has done its work in recent days. Like the breath of God, the Santa Ana winds came up and blew hot. But it was not the Santa Anas that brought the suffering and destruction. It was some human soul that, for reasons beyond imagination, was stirred to strike the match that turned the winds from God's hot breath into a roaring conflagration. When the body was being lifted from the ashes, what did we have to say to those who'd suffered innocently? What do we say to those who loved them, and who want to answer the question "Why?" Love brings a pain no other power can cause.

We need not go so far as the nearby hillsides. Remember the smoke-filled streets of the city, fueled by the anger of injustice and the rage of intolerance. What do we say to the child born to poverty and abuse? What do we say to the father whose little boy is gunned down in some drive-by shooting, to the mother who comes home to a body that was, when she left for work, her three-year-old daughter? Love brings a pain no other injury can deliver.

Thirty years ago this fall, the movement toward freedom for African-Americans—and for all Americans—took a bloody

and memorable turn. The congregation of the Sixteenth Street
Baptist Church had gathered for Sunday school when a bomb,
planted by members of the Ku Klux Klan, exploded, filling the
sanctuary with smoke and blood. We still remember the four
girls who died that day: Addie Mae Collins and Denise McNair,
Carole Robertson, Cynthia Wesley. But what of those who bent
over their shattered bodies? They had suffered fire hoses and
endured beatings, and they sang, "Let freedom ring." Their
clothing had been ripped and their flesh had been torn by the
snarling dogs, and they sang, "We shall overcome." They had
been cursed and spat upon, threatened and denied. But when
they knelt in the ashes, bending over the bodies of the children,
love brought a pain no public torture could match.

I remember the telephone call two years ago that told me I
was on the road to AIDS. My children—Max was three and
Zack was one—were playing a few feet from me. It wasn't possible; I hadn't imagined I was at risk. I stumbled from that
phone call into days and weeks and months of terror. Worst
were the hours I'd see my children sleeping and remember the
virus that was working within me. I'd go to my room and close
the door, shake my fist at heaven, and moan, "If you are God,
and you are good . . . How could you? Where were you when
this happened?" I can understand how Job, or how you, could
be tempted to curse God and die.

But instead of profanity, Job offered praise. In the place of
grief, he clung to grace. "The Lord gave and the Lord has taken
away," he said, "blessed is the name of the Lord."

In the months that followed my diagnosis, I found out where
God was. He was there. He was there more surely than the virus
itself, giving my life new purpose and new meaning, calling me
to a mission I did not want and could not refuse. He was there.

Where was God when the bomb tore apart the bodies of Sunday-school children three decades ago? He was there, in the ashes, waiting to comfort those who mourned; he was there.

Where was God when the towers of flame roared over the hillsides and down through the valleys, consuming the homes and hopes of thousands? He was there, in the ashes, waiting to strengthen those who turned to him; he was there.

And where was God when the city burned in hatred and in fear, when centuries of injustice and decades of indignity broke out in rage and fire. He was there, in the ashes, turning anger to commitment; he was there.

And he is here today, still touching us with comfort, still calling us to commitment, still pressing us toward brotherhood; he is here. Whether we mourn the loss of our homes or hopes, our children or our health, it does not matter; he is here, waiting to whisper comfort when he hears us say: "The Lord gave, and the Lord has taken away; blessed be the name of the Lord."

Across this nation today, one and a half or two million Americans are, as I am, HIV-positive. We are, every one of us, pilgrims on the road to AIDS. We come from every race and culture, every economic and social group. The fastest-growing communities of infection are communities of color, and within them, the rates of infection are growing fastest among women and adolescents. But the virus that eventually pushes us to AIDS doesn't care what color or gender or age we are. It doesn't care if we are homosexual or heterosexual, promiscuous or monogamous, Baptists or Jews. It does not care if our name is John or Betty, Ryan or Arthur, Magic or Mary. To be human is all that's required of these pilgrims on the road to AIDS.

Those of you who've marched for freedom know something about such pilgrims. Some of you are old enough to recall the nights of lynchings and burnings, of flaming crosses and brutal terror. You remember when signs reading NO COLORED were posted—even at the doors of churches. Those who marched for freedom remember the days when, for the sake of your skin color, you were judged less than human. You remember.

Those who are HIV-positive know what it means to be judged less than human. It was not hooded riders who burned to the ground the family's home where children had AIDS; it was their church-going neighbors. But the fire was just as hot and just as angry.

And it was not a county sheriff who stripped naked a young gay man in his locker room and branded the word *AIDS* on his body; it was his high school football team. But the wounds are just as deep, and his mind is just as broken.

And when the pilgrims passed slowly by the church and temple, they did not need to read a sign, NO VIRUS ADMITTED HERE. They'd already heard the message, thundered from a hundred pulpits, that AIDS is "God's judgment." Men on their deathbed, desperate for a taste of God's comfort, have been told that they deserve their disease. Women with AIDS have been treated as if they are guilty and stained, less than human, beyond the reach of God's grace.

We, in the religious communities, took in God's sweet grace and somehow sent out our own mean judgment—as if those who die of heart disease or cancer, or even shootings and bombings, are somehow more loved by God than those who bear my virus.

Those who fueled their march for freedom on the gospel, who walked to the cadence of spirituals and hope, need to come out again and walk with the pilgrim band headed toward AIDS. We are not less than human. You do not contract this disease by loving us or by comforting us or by taking up the cry for justice. When this service has ended, you may avoid me or embrace me; you may shun me or you may hug me—neither can give you AIDS, but one can give me comfort.

When I came to the pulpit this morning, I climbed it in this hope: that some here today would commit themselves to new compassion for those with AIDS. And I will tell you why.

I do not believe that some of us are less than human for the color of our skin or for the virus in our veins, because I believe we are all God's children. Therefore, when justice rolls down like a river, it will wash not only the back of the slave who did not ask for his beating but also the fevered brow of the patient who did not ask for his virus.

I do not believe that the presence of suffering means the presence of guilt, because I remember the suffering of Job, "a blameless and upright man." Therefore, when the healing streams flow through our souls, we will have not judgment but compassion on all those who suffer.

This is what I believe: If you and I both kneel in prayer together, calling one God our Father, how can we not rise and walk together? If—as you lift the shattered bodies of your children and as I fit together the broken pieces of my life—we reach up to touch the hand of the same Father, how can we not see that his children are brothers and sisters? All of us came naked from our mother's womb, and naked we shall return. All of us are children of one Father, members of one broken family searching for one healing.

This is what I believe: You and I cannot call God our Father and deny that we are brothers and sisters. Black or white, HIV-positive or HIV-negative, when we begin our prayers, "Our father who art in heaven," we will end those prayers in the arms of brothers and sisters—else it is not a prayer we offer; it is a lie. This I believe.

This is what I believe: When they drench a man's body in gasoline and send him roaring into flames because he is black, it *is* my brother who runs screaming through the field—because God is our Father. When they exclude a woman from her place in the church, or a child from his place in the school, because of the virus in their veins, it *is* your sister, your child, who cries alone in the night. The lonely man who died of AIDS two blocks from this building this past Thursday night, wondering where God had been; whose brother was he, if not ours? And my children, Max and Zack—whose father died in June, whose mother stands before you now—if my children are not also your children, then whose are they and whose will they be?

In the smoke and rubble that filled this city's streets not long ago, there were those who asked, "Where was God?" If you listen today as AIDS pilgrims march by your sanctuary, you will hear the same question whispered there. The two million Americans headed toward a withering, wasting death are haunted by the question "Where is God?" The time is long overdue for the leadership in our two traditions to step forward. Those who claim to be God's chosen people; those who claim to be washed in God's grace—it is time for us to demonstrate that grace by choosing others as surely as God chose us—by reaching out to those who suffer, by demanding justice, by pouring out compassion, by going into the streets and carrying the pilgrims home to God when they've grown too weak to walk.

Remembering Job's refusal to curse God and die, we sometimes say that someone has "the patience of Job." And I suppose he was a patient man. But, more than patient, I think he was wise. He was wise enough to see that neither tragedy nor poverty nor illness nor grief meant that God had forsaken him—no matter what others came to say.

It is through this wisdom that we can exchange fear for faith. When the test results chill our blood; when everything we've worked to achieve comes crashing down around us; when evil men do evil things to us and those we love—even then, especially then, may we be wise enough to worship in the ashes, saying, "Blessed be the name of the Lord."

Especially in the past few years, as a pilgrim on the road to AIDS, I have come to see that there is no power by which to genuinely forgive, save the power of God. If our hope is going to be placed in ourselves—in the houses we build on the hillsides and the lives we build in our busyness—we will have no refuge when we are left in the ashes. In the quiet that follows the holocaust, it is not the roaring breath of God we hear, but his own still, small voice, speaking through us a word of forgiveness to others, enabling us to turn, rise from the ashes, and say, "Blessed be the name of the Lord."

This congregation has been, for years, a beacon of hope and courage within the Los Angeles community. You have been a living symbol of Job's legacy, encouraging others to bless the name of the Lord. What I ask of you today is this: do not withhold that legacy from pilgrims on the road to AIDS within your community. Reach out with lessons of forgiveness, show them the path to courage, and embrace them with God's grace.

What haunts all of us who are HIV-positive, I think, is the fear that we will not finish. In my last conversation with Arthur Ashe, he worried that he couldn't finish his book *Days of Grace*. My husband, Brian, an artist, worried that he wouldn't finish a canvas he'd begun; after he died, I had the children finish it for him with messages in their favorite colors. And now I worry. Max is six, old enough to know the pain of grief but far too young to bear it well. Zack is four, and full of questions I cannot answer. Like every mother, I want to raise my children to adulthood and watch them launch their own lives of service; I fear that I may not finish. But if there is any lesson to be learned in our two traditions, any truth to be preserved for our children, surely it is this: that God will finish what I cannot complete.

A century and a half ago this morning, the chains of slavery held ancestors to the auction block. Wives were torn from husbands and children from their parents; none could finish what they had begun in love.

A half century ago this morning, the gas chambers were being loaded every hour on the hour in death camps across Europe; what fathers had hoped for their children ended in a shower of final torment, and none could finish what they had begun in love.

"I may not get to the promised land with you," said the Reverend Dr. Martin Luther King Jr. the night before he died, a quarter century ago. He couldn't finish what he had begun in love.

Or . . . did he?

I wish none of our parents had felt the cold chains of slavery or the terror of the death camps; but I am encouraged to believe that, this morning, they may be joined together in a promised land far sweeter than we know. If our lives are truly not our own, but the possession of the God who gave them to us; and if that God is able to help us rise from the ashes of slavery and the death camps—then, perhaps, I can let go of my motherly worries. It may be that I will not finish all that I would like. But, perhaps, both you and I—like those who have gone before us—will finish absolutely everything God has in mind for us.

And when we are finished, you and I, we will rise from the ashes. With all our children, we will rise to see the promise of justice and compassion. And we will say, "Naked I came from my mother's womb and naked shall I return," when we rise.

With our children, we will rise to see the Father who made us one. Young and old, Jew and gentile, we will rise to stand together, and we will say, "The Lord gave, and the Lord has taken away," when we rise.

With all our children, black and white, those we must leave behind and those who've gone before, we will rise from the ashes to see God's kingdom come. And we will say, "Blessed be the name of the Lord," when we rise.

Until we rise together from the ashes, my brothers and sisters, grace to you, and peace.

LOVE AMONG STRANGERS

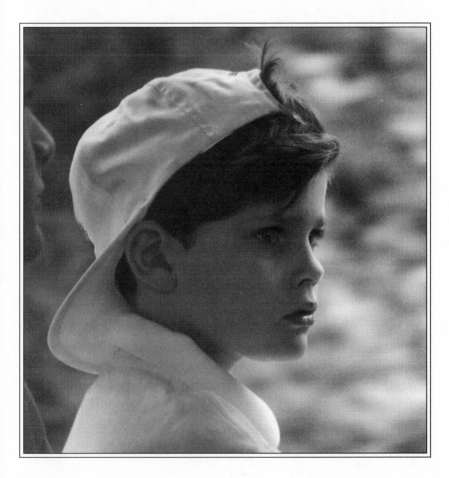

Jeffrey Schmalz Memorial Service
Dalton School
New York City
Tuesday, December 7, 1993

———

I felt so awkward talking to Jeffrey the first time we met. He was the quintessential New York Times *reporter: sophisticated, urbane, analytic. When he wrote notes during our conversations, I worried which evidence of my ignorance he'd just logged.*

How, exactly, we came to love each other is still not clear to me. He was the one I'd call when I needed to understand the policy that made no sense, the turn of events I couldn't imagine. And I was the one he'd call when he was afraid to talk to a group of junior high students at Dalton School. When I heard his soft voice on the telephone, I felt very special.

From his deathbed he had finished his final cover story for the Sunday Times Magazine. *"I have come to the realization that I will almost certainly die of AIDS," he wrote. It was a reality, not a complaint.*

If Jeffrey were still alive, I'd send him this manuscript. I'd say, "Tell me what you think." He'd fax back, "Too many memorial services." And I'd wonder—in the book? or just, too many memorial services?

We first met a little more than one year ago. I was preparing to take on Houston and the Republican National Convention. He was preparing to take on me with an interview at my home.

We began the afternoon as perfect strangers, edgy and cautious. He wanted to know how someone HIV-positive could speak in that place, for those people, for that administration. And so we spoke of politics and priorities while his thin fingers filled his thin reporter's pad with notes. It was nearly dark when we were finishing. He looked away and asked his final question: "Do you sometimes fear dying of AIDS?" I said, "Yes, of course." And when I looked up, I saw his eyes were pools of grief and comfort. He said, "Sometimes I do, too." And we were strangers no more.

One year later, we were together for the last time. The virus was having its way with him. His speech was gone and so I spoke only to his eyes. I sat beside him, telling him that the children were well, and that he had been very brave and that I loved him, and that he could let go now, if he wanted to. In the silence of that room he turned to me and said, in a clear, steady voice, "Your eyes." They were, I suppose, full of grief and, perhaps, comfort.

It was as a man, not a journalist, that Jeffrey first took the measure of AIDS. Young men turned old around him—strong men suddenly groping for their canes to take some feeble step. He knew the long nights of anger, the days of emergency rooms, the failed promise of this week's experimental drug. He knew how bodies could be probed and punctured until all hope was drained from the soul.

And what he knew, he wrote. When presidential campaigns ended and noisy promises were forgotten, his voice grew clearer as he wrote. When we grew angry and took to the streets, expecting at least the satisfaction of one loud scream, Jeffrey wrote in his voice of reason and perspective. When we grew hopeless and took to our beds, hoping at least for the satisfaction of a long-night's cry, Jeffrey wrote with unflinching integrity and not a hint of self-pity. Articulate, balanced, brilliant—story after story, article after article, his voice kept coming even as his strength was fading.

In his final article, he remembered hoping for a cure. "A miracle is possible . . . and for a long time, I thought one would happen. But let's face it, a miracle isn't going to happen. One day soon I will simply become one of the ninety people in America to die that day of AIDS." And so he did. And so we grieve.

But the reason we have gathered at Dalton School has to do not only with grief, but also with comfort. "I cannot imagine addressing a group of high school students," he had told me when I was once extolling the experience. He said he'd been invited here, to Dalton School, but doubted he should come.

I knew what he dreaded. He imagined a room full of young strangers who, hearing his story as a gay man in America, would recoil. He feared that healthy young men would turn away and vibrant young women would fear to be near him. He had tasted rejection before and did not relish tasting it again, in public and on purpose.

Despite his dread, Jeffrey came and stood and spoke in that quiet voice of reason and compassion that makes us long for him tonight. And when he had finished, they did not turn away. They came to him; you, students from Dalton, you came to him with hugs and tears and genuine affection. And we are here to remember not only him, but also you, and the moments you embraced him.

There was no miracle cure. But it may be that another miracle did occur when Jeffrey came to this place—not as a seasoned reporter covering a story but as a vulnerable man telling

the story of his AIDS. Fearing stigma, he found decency; dread-
ing judgment, he found acceptance; doubting himself, he found
love among strangers.

Those of us who are pilgrims on the road to AIDS have not
only lost Jeffrey; we are following him. We praise his courage in
the face of suffering and wonder how we will hold up. We remember his voice of reason in the darkest days, and we wonder
if—when our turn comes—we will feel doubt or anger or some
small grace of comfort. I hear my children cry out in the night
and I wonder what might become of our lives when we all grow
more and more dependent . . . on strangers.

And then I am reminded that we are here, at Dalton School,
because he once came here, too, wondering. Here he found
eyes full of grief and, perhaps, comfort. And who's to say his
mind's eye saw only me when he turned to me one last time to
say, "Your eyes . . ."?

To my fellow pilgrims, in memory of him, I offer this hope:
that when we grow weary and grope for our canes; when our
children grow frightened and grope for some comfort; that we
and they, like Jeffrey, will discover the miracle of love among
strangers.

To all who loved him, and all who mourn—to all who are no
longer strangers—my prayer for healing, with this ancient
promise: grace to you, and peace.

WHEN
WE GROW WEARY

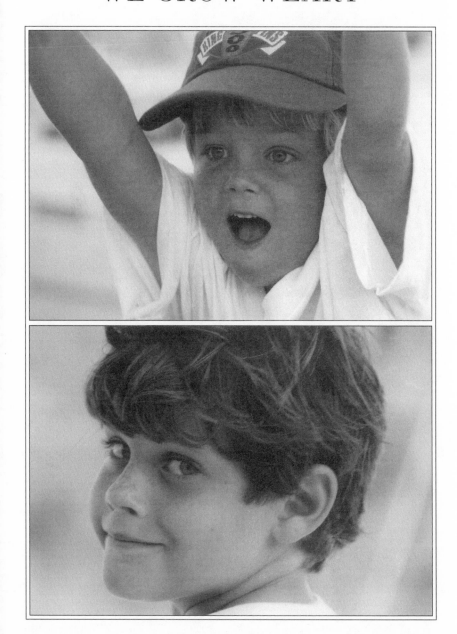

Commencement Address
Self-Taught Empowerment and Pride Program
Rose M. Singer Center
New York City Department of Corrections
Riker's Island, New York
Friday, March 11, 1994

———

On December 11, 1993, I received an honorary doctorate and gave the commencement address at Michigan State University. Fifteen thousand people were in the cavernous arena.

Four days earlier—December 7, the day of Jeffrey Schmalz's memorial—I had gone to the women's prison on Riker's Island to take photographs of caregivers there. I'd expected to uncover some dramatic images for the camera. I'd not expected to discover that I identified completely with the women, especially the HIV-positive women serving sentences. They wondered how long they would live. They worried about their children and who would care for them. I put down my camera and we hugged and we wept and we talked quietly together.

I left Riker's Island in December to tell Michigan State graduates that, "as a mother, so long as I can hear the cry of one child gasping in hunger, my children are not all fed. So long as one African-American man feels the scalding heat of prejudice, my brothers are not all free." That speech came to Michigan from Riker's Island.

And when I went back to Riker's Island on March 11, it was to give another commencement address, this one for the women graduating from the STEP (Self-Taught Empowerment and Pride) Program. No cavernous arena; no cheering crowds. Just women, like me.

T hree months ago, I came to Riker's Island for the first time. I came then as a photographer, planning to take away a series of pictures. But I left as a woman, carrying with me the memories of all those I'd met, including many of you. It was those memories—of the women who hugged me and the stories we shared—that brought me back today with such a sense of honor.

I am honored to be the first to congratulate those who are completing this phase of the STEP Program.

Those of you graduating today have already proven a great deal:

that women who once felt worthless can discover the reality of their own worth—congratulations;

that women who have tasted abuse and addiction can set a course toward wholeness and freedom—congratulations;

that women who felt shame can now raise their heads in dignity; who doubted, now reach for faith; who stumbled, now reach for courage—congratulations.

And I am honored not only to be among you, but also to be one of you. I learned by coming as a photographer that I could not distance myself from you. I could not hide behind a lens or reduce anyone to images I'd come to capture. What I realized profoundly on December 7 is that I am one of us. Like all of you, I am a woman: a daughter, an aunt, a sister, a mother. Like many of you, I am in recovery, clinging to the hope of one more day of clean living. Like some of you, I am HIV-positive, struggling to hold what hope is left.

I was grateful that I could return today to say thank you. Because, when I left three months ago, I took with me some of the strength and courage that I found here. From the woman who told me that she, too, has HIV, I took the certainty that I am not alone; that there are others who understand the fear of losing our children and our lives. From the woman who spoke of years in addiction, and now months in recovery, I took the strength to maintain my own recovery. From the woman who hugged me long and hard and whispered that she would pray for me, I took the hope by which to live "on the outside" for another ninety days. And now I am back, and glad to be with you again.

I did not bring with me a graduation speech adorned with lofty goals and flowery phrases. What I have, instead, is a quiet word or two that I'd like to say, woman to woman, to each of you. I want to say something about tiredness; about wearing down and wearing out; about what we need to do when we grow weary. Because if women who struggle with life know anything, it is this: we will grow weary.

Whether we are graduating today or not, we will grow weary. Whether we are leaving in the coming days or staying, we will grow weary. And if we are to stay the course we've set, if we are to pursue the promises we've made, we must find a way to carry on when we grow weary.

Sometimes we grow weary with the struggle itself. The days grow long and the nights grow longer; a sense of worthlessness steals over us, and we feel lonesome. Soon, we reach out to those who do not love us. We reach for drugs, even knowing they cannot love us. We reach for a bottle, even knowing the bottle will not love us. We reach for a stranger who wants to use us, even knowing he does not love us. But we grow weary of lonesomeness, and we reach out.

Sometimes we grow weary with each other, and we give up. We are mothers of children who would not take guidance and counsel; when they come asking for another chance, we've grown weary of their promises. We are sisters of those who have treated us unkindly; we remember the wounds they inflicted when we were young, the injury that has never healed despite the passing years, and we grow weary. We are daughters who've heard our mother's judgments far too often, and the simple assurance that we are loved far too seldom. We grow weary with each other, and we give up.

Perhaps most often, we grow weary of ourselves. I look for reasons within my life that will give me purpose, and I cannot see them. I listen for answers to those people who judge me harshly for my virus, and I cannot find them. I want to stand up in pride, but I fall down in fear. And I grow weary.

So what shall we do, you and I, when we grow weary? What shall we say to those who want to use us, not love us? What shall we do when we grow weary with each other, and even with ourselves?

This is my suggestion: Let us remember this day and reach out to one another. Let us capture an image in the camera of our minds, caps and gowns, families and friends, and a row of graduates who have proven that—although they have grown weary—they have not given in or given up. Instead, they have reached within for their own worth and reached out to the rest of us for critical support.

When we grow weary on the streets and sidewalks where once we fell; when we are tempted to stumble again; let us remember this day as proof that pride in one's own self can overcome the power of unworthy action. And let us reach out to steady one another.

When we grow weary in our homes and in our families, weary in our cells and in our workrooms, tempted by impatience to give up on one another, let us remember this day as proof that we can take control of our lives—even when we grow weary—if we will support one another.

I've come today not as a photographer, nor as a visitor. I have come as one of you: a woman who knows the taste of terror as well as the promise of hope; a woman articulate about her failings and hard-pressed to name an achievement; a woman in whom good intentions flower, only to wilt when I grow weary. But when I go today, I will take with me the memory of graduates whose lives have been enriched, families whose hopes have been restored, friends and staff whose support has been the root of new pride and new empowerment.

If you see me coming through the door again not long from now, or you meet me in some other setting—do not be surprised. It may only mean that I've grown weary and have come looking for your support. I may have heard another story of families rejecting daughters who have AIDS or read another article on cruel discrimination toward those who are ill. I may have faltered because my children asked hard questions about their father's death or their mother's health, and I could not answer. I may have seen another round of blood tests with dreary results and unsettling numbers, leaving me sleepless and uncertain. If you see me coming, don't be surprised. It only means that another woman, like you, has felt herself growing weary. And she is coming to you—*I* am coming to you—to reach out for support.

My congratulations to those who have achieved graduation. And my thanks for the models of courage and support you have already been in my life.

To you, and to all who grow weary, I offer this promise: If we can remember the power of this day and reach out to steady one another with support, then in the quiet of our weariness we may hear a still, small voice echoing over our lives. And the voice will say: grace to you, and peace.

SPEAK YE COMFORTABLY TO JERUSALEM

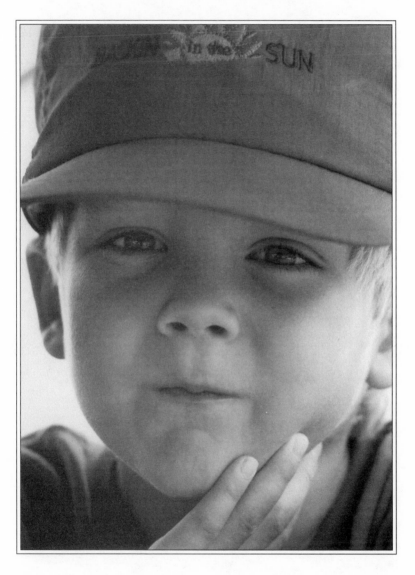

———

During a fall 1993 appearance in a large community center, I'd been surprised by a preteen girl. She'd come up to me after my speech, crying. I presumed she had lost someone or loved someone who was sick. Reaching to hug her, at first I didn't understand what she was saying through her tears. Then I heard her clearly: "It's just so hard, because you can't tell anybody." And I knew: Dawn has AIDS.

I'd preached in Christian churches of nearly all traditions. But this was a rare invitation—from Pittsburgh—to a Jewish temple. It sparked childhood memories of ancient family members intoning holiday prayers. And it helps explain why I chose this place, and these people, to read publicly from Dawn's diary.

As a little girl, when I'd go to temple with my parents, I was so impressed when people came to speak who had written books. I was just awestruck to see and hear them. I could imagine reading books, especially if they had pictures. But I could hardly imagine being so wise, and so important, that I could have produced my own book.

A few months ago my first book, *Sleep with the Angels*, was published—and I was awestruck! I held a copy in my hands the way a mother holds her firstborn. I picked it up and turned it over. I laid it on different tables at the house to see how it looked. I paged through it, amazed to recognize words I'd spoken. And I knew people would read the book, because it has pictures.

But what I wanted most was to go to a temple somewhere—really, like this—and have a libelously exaggerated introduction—like the one I just received. And then I imagined that when I was finished giving a spellbinding speech, you'd parade past tables full of my book, and you'd *ooh* and *aah*, and I'd sit modestly inscribing books for posterity.

So the first thing I did when we arranged to be here was call my publisher. And she called your temple. And then she called me to say, "Temple Sinai doesn't do books."

My people don't do books? A black Baptist church in Atlanta, they had my book; and at a nice Presbyterian congregation in New Jersey, they had my book. I was a very wise Jew in both places—what is this, "My people don't do books?"

At first I thought maybe my people didn't like the book because it has a sermon in it I preached at a California church; then I thought maybe my people just didn't like commerce in temple (even though royalties are contributed to the Family AIDS Network). But then I remembered that on childhood Christmas Eves our Jewish neighbors—who owned Detroit's largest department store—closed late and came home to celebrate the holiday religiously by counting money and singing "What a Friend We Have in Jesus." My people have no fear of Christianity or commerce.

It's fun to tease. Some people imagine that the first symptom of HIV is the loss of a sense of humor. Thank God, that's not true. It isn't possible to live with a four- and a six-year-old and not spend a good deal of time in laughter, often at one's self.

I was surprised, looking back over venues in which I've spoken since early 1992, to discover that this morning is only the second time I've stood before an audience in a temple. Raised in a somewhat recognized Jewish home, I'm not certain how best to account for the fact that I've now preached in a half dozen Christian congregations but this is only my second clean shot at "my people." When I mentioned this to my brother, Phillip, he had two explanations: first, maybe God thought the Presbyterians deserved me, and second, it's always good to practice before the real game. (His sense of humor hasn't diminished either.)

I'm grateful to be with you in this sanctuary today. In the context of a hospice or a caregiver conference, AIDS is a wrenching medical, social, and emotional issue; we ask ourselves how to cope. In the context of a television newscast or a congressional hearing, HIV is a challenge to public policy and personal integrity; we ask ourselves how to prioritize. But in the context of a religious community—when we see something that denies human life and dignity, that yields stigma and suffering—we ask ourselves what we believe. These are questions as deep as our souls. And often we ask them of God, in a single word: "Why?"

When the child in one home is brutalized by a drunken mother while a loving parent next door is struck down by a freewheeling cancer; when a child darts into fatal traffic while an old man lingers hopelessly in a coma; when evil claims the headlines and good is hard to find—before we worship, we're inclined to wonder if God would care to give some answers to our question, "Why?"

Last week, on *Larry King Live,* Mr. King asked me in front of his several million viewers about the impact AIDS has had on "intimacy." He meant, "How's your sex life?" On the way home, I wondered if I really needed to remain a public figure in a public epidemic. On reflection, perhaps I don't so much resent the question as find it uninteresting. A more intriguing inquiry, actually, would have been: How's your spiritual life? What have you learned about the meaning of existence or the purpose of humanity? Do you ever ask yourself, "Why?" or "Why me?" And if you do, what do you have to say?

It was reflecting on those questions, and thinking about seeing you today, that reminded me of the prophet Isaiah. He'd been told by God to speak up, and he wasn't sure quite what to say. "Cry to Jerusalem," said God, and Isaiah responded, "Yes, but, what shall I cry?" And the response, handed down to us in the sacred writings, is a most enduring image:

> Comfort, comfort my people, says your God
> Speak tenderly to Jerusalem, and cry to her
> That her warfare is ended. . . .
>
> He will feed his flock like a shepherd,
> He will gather the lambs in his arms,
> He will carry them in his bosom,
> And gently lead those that are with young.
> *[Isaiah 40:1–2, 11]*

This, of course, is not Jerusalem, and I am not Isaiah. I am an artist and a mother, not a prophet; and your primary concerns probably have more to do with traffic jams and Wall Street jitters than marauding hordes of Philistines. But some of what Isaiah wrestled with in his day, we wrestle with still.

I'm grateful for a family history that runs back to Abraham, for holidays that remind us of our identity. It's good not only for the Jewish tradition, but for all traditions, to know themselves well. Our lives would be dull and gray if not for the gifts of language and dress and history drawn from many groups, each adding the color of its culture and the texture of its tradition. It's good to know who we are.

And it's bad to divide ourselves too sharply from others. Before we begin asserting our identities based on race or gender or religion or nationality, we ought to assert our identities as human beings. For all who claim Abraham as father should go back one more step to Adam, remembering that all men and women are brothers and sisters.

This simple idea—as acceptable as motherhood and apple pie—has emerged from some painful, recent experience. For more than two years I've crisscrossed the nation pointing to indisputable realities and issuing reasonable warnings. And I regret to report that I've been nicely received—warm smiles, generous ovations, and affectionate pats on the head—by people who, as they climbed into their cars to go home, said to each other, "Isn't it awful about those people? I feel so bad for them."

I've known for some years the power of denial, but I never knew it as potently as I know it now. We study the demographics of the epidemic together until I hear him say, "Well, I'm not on the chart—it can't be me." One, maybe two million Americans are infected, and we conclude, "Thank God it's not my children; they're all straight." We cling to myths no longer true, if they'll bolster our denial. We'll forget our own moments of risk; we'll redefine the categories to keep ourselves out. "I'm married," she said; "I'm a mother; I'm not that kind of woman. It couldn't, possibly, be me."

I know about being married, and being a mother, and not being what others call "that kind of woman." I know it all quite well. I also know that somewhere between one and two million Americans are infected today. And the leading cause of their infections was the conviction that it couldn't, possibly, be them.

When a stable sense of identity becomes a smug sense of security; when we're sure that, because of who we are, because of the group that surrounds us, we are beyond risk—these are the moments we're speeding toward very grim moments in this epidemic. Being Jewish is no protection from AIDS; neither is being nice or wealthy or skilled at denial.

There is no community insured by God against calamity. It's hard to imagine that between the lines parading into *Schindler's List* and those coming out of the Holocaust Museum, any Jewish congregation would deny that bad things can happen to good people. But we are not exempt from this remarkable conclusion.

When first I went public, I'd occasionally rail against the fundamentalist preacher who pounded his airwaves' pulpit and raged against "the sin of sodomy," which God was "punishing with AIDS." Frankly, the number of people who hold to that heresy is quite small—it's a mean group, but a little one.

But I'm amazed at the number of people who casually regard success as a sure sign of God's blessings, and life challenges as some indication that God may be up to something other than love. This is a dangerous notion, more dangerous than fanatics who haunt late-night airwaves to raise money for their crusades. Because this idea, once firmly implanted, leaves those who suffer with the latent fear that, really, their suffering is self-induced. If they'd been better people, they'd be "blessed," too—and they'd not suffer.

I was shooting photos at an AIDS housing program called Stand Up, Harlem, a month or two ago. A group of young, HIV-positive women were talking about their families and the rejection they felt. One beautiful woman, perhaps twenty years old, finally said, "I wish I had cancer instead of AIDS. I could stand the treatments and the pain and my hair falling out. And I'm going to die anyway. But then, at least, my family wouldn't reject me. I could go home."

Is there a moral difference between one virus and another?

Why would we stiff-arm a daughter with AIDS while embracing a daughter with cancer? I fear the answer is this: despite our loud rejections of fundamentalist TV screamers, we hold their beliefs, only more quietly. We think of AIDS as something earned, as if those who carry the virus made a wasting death their goal and have now achieved it.

This is an ugly notion, as old as the Book of Job: the idea that when life is sleek and easy, we're rolling around in blessings, and when life grows grim and hard, the blessings are no longer there.

I'm convinced, based on my experience and that of thousands I've met, that grief can be the instrument by which we come to grace; that sickness can be the vehicle we ride to new depths of self-discovery or charity toward others; that pain and loss and grueling anxiety can be the pathway by which we come to a rock-hard certainty about our own purpose. Of course it isn't the pathway I'd choose; but we don't make the choices. And we'd be wise to take a cautious view of what's a blessing and what's not, remembering what I believe is an old Dutch proverb: "God sometimes strikes straight with a crooked stick."

This is, I think, the third time in little more than two years that—in a public setting—I've quoted the same words from the prophet Isaiah. The last time was at the memorial service for Brian, the man with whom I shared a marriage and two children and one virus. I cited it there, in a context of many faiths, because I saw it pointing to a single source of comfort.

The first time I read these words was at a service of healing and remembrance, in the sanctuary of a tiny stone church in rural North Carolina. We'd gone there not only for the service, but to pay our respects to the priest who was leading it. In the early days of the epidemic he had been told to refuse Communion to those who carried the virus; in response, he gave them a special place at the Communion rail and carried the sacrament to their bedsides. He was told that if he invited people with AIDS into his home, it would be burned; he turned his home into a hospice. When local morticians refused to embalm a young man who'd died of AIDS, he said the dead had no need of morticians, but the living have great need of compassion.

In the annals of the AIDS epidemic, some religious communities and leaders have been exemplary, models not only of decency but of heroism. And some have not. The Jewish community has, as nearly as I can tell, reflected this pattern as well. In some quarters we've made outstanding contributions, and in others we've made no contribution at all. Regrettably, the annals of this epidemic appear to be far from closed—and there is great room for Jewish communities to assume roles of leadership and contribution.

And the need is not hard to identify; sometimes it is as simple as the child next door.

Last fall our work was the focus of an ABC *Nightline* special with Ted Koppel. One of the events covered by the film crew was a speech I gave to a community group. At the close of the speech that evening, I'd left the stage to meet people, and—completely unrehearsed and unexpected—the camera and microphone caught me embracing a child of eleven whose name, I later discovered, was Dawn. She and her mother were both crying as they came up to me, and when I reached out to comfort Dawn with a hug, I—and the microphone—heard her say, "It's just so hard, so hard not to be able to tell somebody." She had AIDS, and her family had warned her against letting others know the truth because there is no way to speak comfortably about this disease.

In the months that followed, Dawn and her parents visited our home in Washington, D.C., when Dawn was in town for treatment at NIH, the National Institutes of Health. On perhaps their second visit, she brought a copy of a diary she'd been keeping. And this is one of the entries:

When you live with HIV there are . . . good days. Going to the mall with my good friend who knows my diagnosis is fun because this is a day when I don't have to worry about what I say. This is also one of the only days where I don't have to hide in a bathroom to take my medicine. . . .

There are definitely bad days, too. These are the days when the kids talk about AIDS in school and about how they would never touch or go near kids who have it. I once asked a boy what he would do if I had it, and he told me he would never go near me, but that he knew I didn't really have it. He was wrong. I do. And I do have bad days where a lot of things hurt like my legs, my head, my stomach, my ears. . . .

The most difficult days are when I can't help but think a lot about if I am ever going to get cured. Sometimes . . . I think I am not. . . .

It is just very hard coming back to NIH when you know that if you make a friend he may die. My best friend here died. I get scared. . . . So sometimes I just get real quiet and stick to myself.

When I hear Dawn's soft agonies, I cannot help but wonder what Max will write when he arrives at eleven, five years from now. And Zack, who's now a fully energized four-year-old— what quiet corner will he find in which to hide?

This is my appeal to you: that those of us within secure families and comfortable communities, who meet within a long tradition of worship and hope, give up our own hiding places. This is not somebody else's disease, if we are truly brothers and sisters in a single family. We do not need to wait until the virus is in our bloodstreams to act. You can educate now, call for compassion now, break down walls and stereotypes and cruelties now. At one extreme, there are national priorities to challenge; at the other, there's a local hospice in which the breathing stops on a regular basis. There's work to be done by people who have a firm and rooted integrity, and who live with the conviction that we are human.

Perhaps I was once too timid to challenge bigotry and stigma, even when I saw it taking a toll, too quiet to raise my voice against intolerance, too comfortable to launch a volley against complacency. I do not know what's changed me most, my boys or the disease. But I can tell you that I have grown passionate about the values of my community and yours, because my children may need to live in it. I will invest hours doing what I can to shape their conscience at home; but they will have years at the mercy of the consciousness of communities in which they mature. And they will learn what others have to teach them.

And in the harder stretches of the day, or night, it is here that I find comfort in a community of faith. Those who genuinely believe that God has called them to do his work are a great hope. Because it is they who are likely not merely to hear Isaiah's words, but to act on them.

I do not live my life waiting to die. But if I am to live hopefully, I must do it with the confidence that should I no longer be able to carry on, my children will be carried on without me. When they are hungry for affection and comfort, someone needs to feed them. When they've fallen and are bleeding, someone needs to pick them up. When they are broken by grief, as we all are from time to time, someone needs to carry them gently.

If it is God's work, then it is fitting work for his people. And I take hope in the promise that you will step forward in that day. It is not so impossible a task. You need only to feed my children like a shepherd, gather them like lambs into your arms, carry them cradled in your bosom, and lead them gently into comfort.

Until that day, grace to you, and peace.

IGNORANCE
IS THE ENEMY

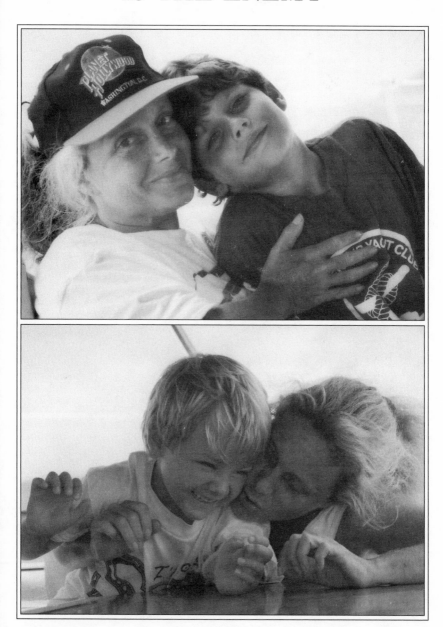

Unique Lives & Experiences Lecture Series
Toronto, Ontario
Monday, May 9, 1994

———

So who'd have ever imagined that I'd be on the public lecture circuit, playing to a packed house in Toronto, filling the open slot between Candice Bergen and Shirley MacLaine?

Unique Lives & Experiences is Canada's most famous public lecture series. I'd never heard of it, of course, in part because I'm not Canadian and in part because I'd never been a public lecturer. So I was a little surprised when we received the invitation.

I was on my way to the hall when someone read the press release about the event. According to the release, the evening's speaker was going to be "riveting" and "unforgettable." I could hardly wait to hear her.

Visualize this: you're trying to put on lipstick in the back-seat of a bouncing car, after a bedtime telephone call to two children who are hysterical because their mother has gone to another country, and—just as you realize you're wearing shoes of two different colors and your dress has a wad of bubble gum stuck to the hem—you hear the press release promise

*that the evening's speaker will, and I quote, "stun you by her
beauty and courage."*

*I told the audience, later, what I actually thought: "Forget
beauty; just showing up takes courage."*

I was asked to speak this evening under the title "Ignorance Is
the Enemy." The assumption embedded in this title is that, if
we knew more about AIDS, we would do more about AIDS. And
I may as well tell you at the beginning that I am not sure this is
true.

The biological facts of AIDS are widely known. The disease
is transmitted by an exchange of bodily fluid in which the virus
is concentrated, typically blood or semen. You can pick it up
from sex but not from sneezes, from needle exchanges or blood
transfusions—but not from a child's hug or a lover's tears.

The medical facts are equally clear. As nearly as we can tell,
the cure rate on AIDS is zero and the kill rate is 100 percent.

Because HIV is transmissible, AIDS is an epidemic growing
exponentially on both sides of the border. I've never really
known why governments report cases of AIDS instead of numbers of infections, but I've never believed they do so out of ignorance. About a third of a million AIDS cases have been
reported in North America. That's alarming. Even more alarming is that we have at least one million infections, all headed toward AIDS, and underreporting is significant. Perhaps it isn't
true that one million of us are HIV-positive. Perhaps two million of us are.

Because AIDS can develop slowly and without immediate
symptoms, hundreds of thousands of North Americans are infected today who do not know it. They've never been tested. For
them, it *is* true that ignorance kills. They're unlikely to extend

their lives with medical support because they don't know they need it. But they're likely to extend the epidemic by transmitting the virus to others. And so, while you and I visit here this evening, another one or two dozen North Americans will pick up the virus and start down the road to AIDS.

But is it really ignorance that keeps alive the myth that this is a disease of homosexuality, largely confined to gay communities? Last year in North America, the majority of sexual transmissions were heterosexual, and within those transmissions, the majority of persons becoming infected were women. The fastest-growing rates of infection in North America are among heterosexual young adults and women. Is it ignorance that resists this information?

Medically, scientifically, empirically—it's clear that this is a disease of people—not gay people or poor people or people of color or people of sin—just people. Like you and me.

But, personally, what's not very clear is the role that ignorance plays. I used to believe if people knew better, they'd behave better. But I'm no longer so sure. And I'll tell you why.

I discovered nearly three years ago that I am also on the road to AIDS. I am no longer a spectator; I'm a traveler. When I asked others on the road to AIDS how I could help, they said, "Tell your story to those we can't reach. Go to the suburbs and to the families; go to the straight communities and to the women. Tell them, show them, that this is their disease."

And so I took my story on the road. From the country churches of North Carolina to the college campuses of Utah, from living rooms in Memphis to hospices in Grand Rapids, from the Senate of Puerto Rico to the center of Amsterdam—I mounted pulpits and lecterns and spoke to them of AIDS. I called for awareness, I asked for compassion, and I challenged those not yet infected to act.

And they applauded me warmly and they thanked me kindly and they went home convinced it "could not happen here." I said, "Look at me," and they nodded wisely; I said, "Look at your children," and they hugged them closely. They took refuge in a blindness I cannot cure, a denial I cannot break.

Last week in a high school in Illinois I moved a fourteen-year-old to uncontrollable tears. Weeping, she came backstage to read her Bible to me lest I should go to hell. What she'd heard was not that she was at risk, but that I was; she feared not for her life, but for my eternal welfare. It isn't that I failed to understand her love for me. What concerns me is that my message did not convince her; my story did not change her. Someone must tell me how to do it differently, because I've gone on the road, and I've gone home . . . discouraged, and uncertain that ignorance is really the enemy.

We need to educate. Children must be taught. Silence on this topic is deadly and cowardly and wrong. But it is not only ignorance that it is the enemy; it is denial.

I stand before an audience of married people and tell them I became infected in marriage. But the myth is so powerful that this is a gay disease or a distant disease or someone else's disease, that their denial takes over before my reality sinks in.

I see an audience of women and don't know how to move them, how to convince them—convince you—that the threat is tangible and real. Do I tell my story of being a married woman again? Do I show charts? Cite statistics? Is there something here that I am missing, that contributes to the ignorance?

I doubt it. Slowly, somewhat sadly, but quite surely, I have come to believe that—while ignorance is a danger—denial is the greater killer. For those who contracted the disease a decade ago, I can easily believe they did not know. But for those who incur the risks today, I can hardly imagine it.

There comes a time when we can no longer say, "I didn't know." The time has arrived when truth would say, "I would not listen. I did not want to hear."

But truth itself is sometimes clouded, and that is also worth a moment of our time.

Within our communities, the moral standards are largely determined by people like you and me, people with influence and stature—men in high-rise offices and women in high-powered clubs; people with good educations and nice homes, who go to temple on Friday and church on Sunday and make decisions about what is acceptable, and what is not.

We are responsible for the moral character of our homes, our businesses, our communities. Our community's moral fabric does not just happen; we make it happen. We weave it from our attitudes and behaviors. We define who will be praised and who will be shunted to the side, who will be lauded in the social pages of the local paper and who will be mocked in our private jokes. We decide who is touchable, and who the untouchables will be, in our society.

And those with AIDS have, in community after community, become the untouchables. They've been isolated and despised. I've held weeping children who dared not tell anyone of their diagnosis. I've listened to parents describe suffering their children endured at the hands not of the virus but of the neighborhood. I've met young adults who confessed to their families that they'd contracted the virus and were—for their confession—evicted from their family homes.

The infection strikes, eventually the symptoms show up, the test is taken, the news is delivered, and we are face-to-face with our mortality. Then comes the decision: to tell or not to tell.

If we have cancer, we tell and others rally to our support. If we have coronaries or strokes, we tell, expecting sympathy if

not support. But if we have HIV, we are quiet, uncertain, waiting for the stigma and discrimination to begin.

How do we account for this? Why would someone with a
virus expect to be marked for prejudice and treated to abuse?
Why would they fear? The answer, I'm afraid, is simple: they
have seen our communities at work. Despite our progressive
ideals and our liberal campaigns, they've seen that we treat
AIDS not as a virus, but as a moral failure. We do not really believe that AIDS is like the flu and the common cold, striking
both bishops and thieves without evidence of either innocence
or guilt.

We've forgotten that the virus has no moral value. Or, worse,
we've forgotten that we do—that you have moral value, and I
do. It is morality, as much as medicine, that has failed us.

For women, the environment of judgment and discrimination
is especially bitter. We as mothers contend with our death in
the face of our children's continuing lives and needs. When
funds are limited and choices must be made, many mothers invest in their children's health—letting their own slide away.
When neighbors are vicious and judgments are likely, mothers
choose to hide their HIV status to protect their children from
the taunts of playmates and the outright cruelties of adults.

But it goes deeper than that, even if we rarely admit it.
Women are raised in a society that says we should be pristine
and beautiful, wonderfully groomed and tastefully modest. If we
would like companionship and intimacy, we must pass the test
of worthiness. Then comes the diagnosis. And the culture that
has raised us delivers yet another message to us. You who are
infected are neither tasteful nor modest; you are wanton
women. You are not pristine; you are dirty women. You have
failed the test of worthiness. You are untouchable.

These messages were first delivered to gay men, who did not

deserve them, and are now being delivered to infected women, who do not deserve them either.

The morality that stands behind such ugly judgmentalism is, in fact, immorality. It is not decency; it is indecency.

But when we walk the winding hallways of the Holocaust Museum, we embrace the idea of *evil*. When the Ku Klux Klan rallies and we smell burning crosses; when the homes of children with AIDS are reduced to smoking rubble; when we hear MPs wishing to block an international conference of HIV-positive people, or dying men told that God delights in their suffering—no explanation short of evil is very satisfying.

And evil must be confronted. A century ago in the American South, as the battle over slavery was about to break into civil war, an ex-slave named Frederick Douglass spoke clearly about those who see the moral struggle but do not want to confront it. They are, he said, "men who want crops without plowing the ground. They want rain without thunder and lightning. They want the ocean without the awful roar of its many waters. The struggle may be a moral one or it may be a physical one or it may be both moral and physical. But it must be a struggle. Power concedes nothing without a demand. It never did and never will."

Ignorance is no doubt an enemy. But immorality is a greater enemy by far. And I am here, tonight, to ask that you join me in the opposition. We need leaders unafraid of those who cheer on cruelty, undeterred by those who call for bigotry and hatred. We need heroes who have no fear of embracing an infected woman, no hesitancy in taking the hand of a dying man to assure him that he has value. We need *un*infected people who will reject the pious judgments of self-righteous people and embarrass them with a model of compassion.

I recognize that I am asking you to take a risk, but I have no choice. We need some of you willing to risk careers and social positions, believing that a life of integrity brings wealth that cannot be purchased during a good day on Wall Street. We need corporate executives from Yonge Street convinced to their bones that anything less than compassion is unworthy, home-makers from Burlington persuaded that anything short of jus-tice is unacceptable. We are hungry for moral leadership—and those who shape their communities' standards could provide it.

And before I leave this appeal, let me ask that those of you who are uninfected not only join the struggle but stay with it. Those of us already infected have no choice. Over and over I've told audiences that I am no hero, that I didn't take on my role in this matter willingly—I was drafted, I did not enlist, and I de-test the virus that put me here.

But, wherever we are, we are called to do the right thing, even when doing the right thing doesn't "work." We take a strong moral stand; our business partners call us a fanatic. We reach out to help someone whose life has fallen to pieces; for our charity, we're lied to and cheated by the person we've aided. We work day and night, exhausting ourselves on behalf of a woman in need—and when we're finished, she dies. Some-times morality doesn't "work."

But morality is not measured by effectiveness; it is measured by rightness. Christians at Calvary and Jews at Auschwitz can plainly see that the truth may not always "work," but it is still truth. We do what is right, not because it works, but because it is right. Join the struggle, and do not leave it.

A year ago, perhaps to the day, the man from whom I con-tracted the virus became terribly ill. Brian wanted to see the boys again, and we traveled to see him. What happened in the following month was life-changing for me. As the fevers grew and the end became undeniable, we remembered together the times before the anger pulled us apart.

As we approached his final days, I realized that I was unprepared and frightened to be with someone at death's door. I had never been so intimate with death and dying. I didn't know what to expect or what to do or even what to say. I did not feel moral or heroic; I felt terrified, helpless at the thought of being at his bedside when he died.

What I learned as Brian died is that one doesn't really need to do very much; being there is adequate, demonstrating by your presence that they are not alone. No special words are called for in the final moments. I think there was a quiet "I love you," and perhaps one whispered "I'll miss you," and finally a gentle "It's enough, Brian, let go."

All our years of education, every dollar we've earned and saved, each trophy we've mounted, each headline we've grabbed—in the end, what we want is what we've wanted all along: someone to touch our hand and tell us we are loved. And what we have to offer is nothing more, or less, than ourselves.

I was pulled away from Brian's bedside an hour after his struggle had ended. To be perfectly candid, I think I envied his passing. Seeing what the virus could do, I did not want to take on the future. But, it was not my time. And there were the children.

Some months later I was reading a book that many women found inspiring, *Women Who Run with the Wolves*. And it occurred to me that perhaps one thing I could do is be more bold in speaking as a woman to other women.

The issue faced by women uniquely involves our own sense of power, or lack of it; our willingness to reach out in boldness, or our inability to do it. We stake our happiness and our sense of self-worth on relationships that are fragile, even dangerous. We find ourselves alone with someone we love, and we're stunned when we receive not affection but abuse. We dare not challenge someone who seems stronger; we dare not stand up, either to fight or to flee. And so we vacillate between disbelief and terror, uncertain whether the fear of being left alone is greater than the fear of dying. In truth, the question we're avoiding is, "What's our life worth?"

I was thinking about this when I read: "Afraid to stop, afraid to act, repeatedly counting to three and not beginning . . . these become epidemic anywhere and anytime women are captured. . . . A healthy woman is much like a wolf: robust, chock-full, strong life force, life-giving, inventive, loyal, roving. We are not meant to be puny with frail hair and inability to leap up, inability to chase, to birth, to create a life."

Here was an image of women who are bold and courageous, a clear demand to challenge women who leave themselves in harm's way to maintain either their self-image or their dependencies. And then the author went on:

> I once dreamt that I was telling stories and felt someone patting my foot in encouragement. I looked down and saw that I was standing on the shoulders of an old woman who was steadying my ankles and smiling up at me.
>
> I said to her, "No, no, come stand on *my* shoulders for you are old and I am young."
>
> "No, no," she insisted, "this is the way it is supposed to be."
>
> I saw that she stood on the shoulders of a woman far older than she, who stood on the shoulders of a woman even older, who stood on the shoulders of another. . . .
>
> This is the way it is supposed to be. The nurture for telling stories comes from those who have gone before. . . .

And so I've gone back on the road to tell my story, hoping some young man will hear more clearly than I can say that I would like to save his life, wishing that some young woman whose self-esteem has been crushed will not place herself in harm's way for the sake of one night of comfort.

I've hoped that by telling my story, someone who has been at risk might get strong and get tested; that a community dressed out in attitudes of meanness and stigma might discover a moral decency rooted in compassion and dignity; that a lonely woman, asking herself, "What's my life worth anyway?" might hear not only my voice, but God's, saying, "You are worthy, and your life is worth my own."

And the story is not yet finished. Because I can now go home to tell my children stories about you. They have looked down the road their father took; sometimes they look at me, wondering how far down that road their mother has gone. We don't know that, but we know enough: someday, probably too soon, I'll grow weary and, like all the pilgrims on this road, need to lay down to rest. But the story I bring home from Toronto could be a great comfort. If you would join the campaign for compassion, I can tell first-grader Max—who yesterday lost his first tooth—that he will someday see you coming down the road behind us, willing to take his hand. If you would challenge the stigma and discrimination, then it would be easy for me to offer you as hope to four-year-old Zack.

If you have now become part of my story, I can assure my children that, when the hard day comes, you will be there, teaching them how to say "I love you," letting them know it's okay to say "I'll miss you," helping them help me to finally let go.

I'll go home to tell Max and Zack that some good people I met in Toronto will drop by someday when most they're needed. Until then, grace to you, and peace. Good night.

THE WAY THINGS ARE

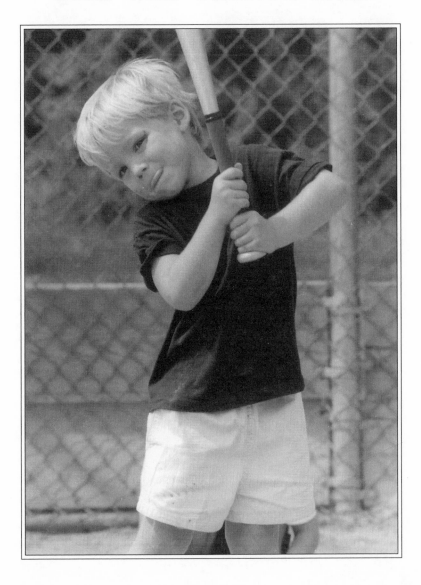

Sotheby's
New York City
Wednesday, June 8, 1994

————

Somewhere between the close of the Eisenhower era and the opening of the Kennedy presidency, my father was divesting himself of the oil business that he had turned into a success by every measure. In the years that followed—at an age equated by some to a word he does not understand, retirement—*he distinguished himself as a philanthropist, a presidential adviser, and a corporate board member.*

One of the businesses in which he has maintained both an ownership and a personal interest is the world-famous "auction house" named after its British founders: the Sotheby's.

When the chief executive officer of Sotheby's said that she wanted to raise HIV consciousness among her staff colleagues and wondered if I would speak at an after-hours reception, I was delighted. It gave me an opportunity to blend my family history with my personal passion.

What I had not anticipated was how difficult it would be, how vulnerable I would feel, telling the truth in this place.

I remember visiting Sotheby's when I was somewhat younger, wondering what I might do with the rest of my life. Seeing the works of the masters as they came through your hands, I remembered that Rembrandt had nearly frozen to death watching wives and children die in poverty, that van Gogh had chopped off one ear and most of his sanity before his early death, and that others had suffered awful horrors while giving the world their art.

After considering all these things—I said to myself, "I think I'll be an artist!"

I don't know precisely what that says about my grasp on reality. But it may remind us that things are not always quite as they seem. The private and human realities are often very different from the public and enduring images we create. I think I've learned this simple reality—that things are not always as they seem—at the loss of considerable innocence.

I was raised in a family that did not let prejudice through the doors, at least not if it was blatant; and so I grew up believing that stigma or hatred were not alive or well in my community. I was schooled in a context where justice seemed to flow down for all, so I didn't expect that injustices were commonplace in the lives of others. I'd heard of anti-Semitism and knew that my father fought it; I'd heard of racism and imagined that we were not guilty of it. Raised in a genteel moral silence, I was amazed when cries of injustice ignited city streets and echoed through my early adulthood. Things were not as I had thought; not at all.

I was raised in a context of fatherly excellence. My father is a wise man, widely loved—also by me. But I was not raised with the expectation that I would be wise or widely respected. That was my father's calling. And whether we grow in a context of abuse or of affluence, the context itself does not give us a sense of calling or of self-worth. It could not teach me the value of me or enable me to believe that I was gifted. Measuring myself against the standard of his success, I could only see the ways in which I failed.

And so I'd come to Sotheby's, quietly longing to be some unknown artist: not someone's daughter, but me. I wanted to be known for production, not pedigree; for creativity, not club membership. I'd never frozen in an Amsterdam studio. I'd kept both of my ears and some of my sanity. My studios have always been compulsively neat and unbelievably organized. But, despite all that, I wanted to be a real artist. Only now, years later, can I look back to see that things are not always as they seem.

And neither are we. Being a union member does not make you a thug, being an antiquities expert does not make you a bore, and being a Republican does not make me immune. We are quick with our assumptions, agile with our labels, gifted at our judgments, and deadly in our errors.

It's often hard for us to tell the truth about ourselves. How many years have some of us spent avoiding the simple sentence we finally learned to say: "My name is Mary, and I'm an alcoholic"? How many family secrets have we kept? How many brutal moments have we repressed? We are not always as we seem, even to each other.

And so we gather in this magnificent hall, where treasures of the world have traded hands, to discuss in polite terms and civil expressions an epidemic that has already claimed several hundred thousand American lives. At least one, perhaps nearly two million Americans have been infected with HIV; all are on the road to AIDS, some closer to the beginning of that road, others nearly at its end. This year, more Americans will fall in the fight with AIDS than fell over nine years in Vietnam; next year, the number will be greater.

Things are not always as they seem. And in a terribly important sense, in the face of the most deadly epidemic in human history, it is not AIDS that we need to discuss. We must talk about ourselves.

We can draw charts and show slides; we can point to demographics and beg for new policies—but the truth is, the virus is having its way with us and with our children. And if we are to endure this epidemic, it is not the virus that must be changed first; it is we.

A year ago I visited an exclusive girls school in this city. I went at the request of my doctor, whose daughter attends there. On my first visit, I met with the students. Then I went back to meet with parents and staff. In the second meeting, after I'd spoken, parents asked polite questions and staff expressed their sympathies. Until an eleventh-grade student, who'd helped organize the event, asked to report briefly on a confidential questionnaire completed by students.

I think the breathing actually stopped in that room when she said, "The seventh- and eighth-grade girls want to know how they can get tested for HIV . . . anonymously." Suddenly parents didn't want a biological explanation of the virus; they wanted to know if their daughters had been surveyed. A staff member asked if she might be at risk. We stopped talking about a virus and began talking about ourselves.

Some people remember that I spent thirteen minutes in Houston a few years ago talking to some Republicans. But for sheer satisfaction, if you would like to come with me into genuinely moving conversations, I would take you not to a well-lit stage in the Astrodome but to the dimly lit bowels of Riker's Island, to the shadowy room where we held hands to remember those who had died; to the prison nursery, where children of HIV-positive women give them a reason to live; to the chaplain's office where we wept together and prayed together and recommitted our lives together.

Or come with me to the gay community where women and men, black and brown and white, gave up looking for justice or longing for compassion and became healers of one another. Watch a man sit up all night, bathing a lover's open sores, knowing he is looking at his own future. It's easy to speak hopefully of a cure at a conference; try whispering that optimism at an AIDS hospice in the gay community. It's easy to speak of human goodness at a cocktail party; try it sometime near the gates of Dachau.

Things are not always as they seem. But in a community where values are sound, surely we would go to those who are dying and say, "Let us hold you." In a nation where values are corrupt, we might go to the dying and say, "Let us judge you." On this criterion alone, the values of the gay community are worthy not only of our praise, but of our imitation.

Let me say this as plainly as I can: the virus is deadly. But so is ignorance. So is prejudice. So is hatred. Fear and intimidation and judgmentalism are weapons as dangerous, as capable of destroying us all, as the nuclear weapons we've wanted to set aside. We worry about the virus, and I am glad. I only wish we worried as much about values. We die by the virus, but we live by the values we hold: whether we embrace those different from ourselves or hate them. Whether we rush to cradle the injured, lift the sick, comfort the grieving—or whether we carefully insulate ourselves from all the gritty agonies, all the human tragedy, that can turn us nauseous or teach us nobility. The virus frightens us; but some values should terrify us.

I moved to Washington last year and enrolled my children, one in a private and the other in a public school. Because I assumed that things were as they seemed, I was concerned about how things would go in the public school—whether Max would have to wrestle with stigma or name-calling because his mom is HIV-positive (and public about it).

But things are not always as they seem and I was not yet prepared for the quiet prejudices and ugly behaviors that are covered by generous contributions to fashionable causes.

Things are not always as they seem, and neither are we. But that's really not my point this afternoon. This is: we can change the way things are. We can make changes in our lives, in our relationships.

It's an enormous irony that the virus that may kill me has enabled me to examine, and in some respects to change, my life. I'm still Mary Fisher, still not so certain of my value and gifts, still frightened by the thought of an especially vicious critic having at my art. But, struggling with the virus, I've learned something about our ability to change.

I've learned the limits of sympathy, as wonderful as sympathy may be. I give a speech and a thousand people file by me to say they wept and tell me that they care. I'm grateful for their sympathy. But what I want—and what they need to stay alive— is action. And I am terrified when I see that an audience was moved to weep in the auditorium, but not to act in their everyday lives.

I've learned that I can be very angry, despite discomfort with my anger, and that anger—like sympathy—has limits.

Anger comes when friends die. I was angry when Arthur Ashe died. I was angrier still when Jeffrey Schmalz died. I was angriest of all when I realized how few people really cared that either had come or gone. Even though they were famous, one was black and one was gay—and, to be brutally truthful, that had made a difference. I am angry that we have not valued lives enough to save them, in part because the lives belonged to gay men or poor women, to those who are African or Asian or something other than we are. I am angry that someone would think my life is more worthy than theirs because I contracted a virus in marriage, or that someone would think my life is less worthy because I contracted it at all. My God, what are we doing to each other with these judgments?

I was angry that my husband, however unknowingly, played fast and loose with my life, and my children's lives. I was angry when he told me I needed to be tested, and when the results rolled in. But my anger could not repair our relationship, only forgiveness could do that. And when he died in my arms, I had a lot of feelings. Anger was not one of them.

Anger and sympathy are both to be expected. But neither is enough. We must find a way to move from our emotions to our commitments, from our momentary feelings to our reliable behaviors. And we must find a way to do it together—because, alone, we cannot survive, let alone make the changes that are needed.

I don't know what changes to expect of Sotheby's. I don't expect Sotheby's to find a cure; but I would be heartened if Sotheby's were a model of compassion for other institutions. I would be grateful if you focused not merely on the virus that can kill us, but on the values that can redeem our lives and make us worthy. I'd be proud to read in some annual report not only about the bottom line of profit, but also about the consequence of moral commitment. I'd love my association with a corporation that valued people for what they are: people. Black people or white, male or female, straight or gay, immigrant or native born, in sickness and in health . . . people. That is my hope for you.

And for my children, who may one day come to Sotheby's as I once did. My greatest fear, of course, is not that they will fail to learn about the great artists of the world, but that—should I be gone—the world will fail to teach them about love and compassion. The world will teach them plenty about judgment; but, if I am gone, who will teach them about grace? Perhaps, Sotheby's? Perhaps . . . you?

Until the day my children come calling on Sotheby's, grace to you, and peace.

FOR THE
GENERATION STILL TO COME

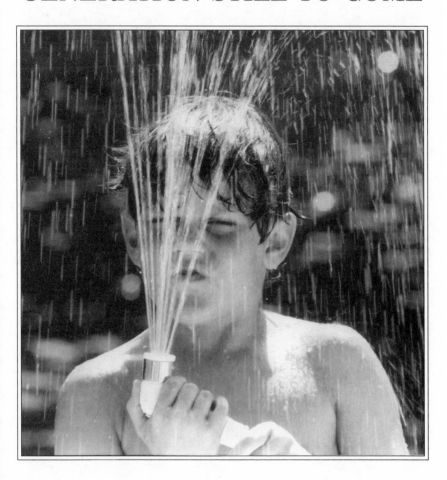

FDA Blood Products Advisory Committee
Hearing on Home-Access HIV Testing
Washington, D.C.
Wednesday, June 22, 1994

———

Johnson & Johnson took on a corporate venture known as Di-rect Access Diagnostics to design, produce, market, and sell an HIV home-access testing service. The idea was simple: people would buy an inexpensive kit, take a small blood sample at home, send in the sample, and receive results and counseling privately by telephone. If additional counseling was required, people would be connected to professional staff. Quality control was immaculate. The concept was flawless. And the United States government said, "No . . . this needs more study."

We have no cure for AIDS and no effective preventative. We can initiate life-prolonging treatments only if we know who is HIV-positive. The majority of the one to two million Americans who are positive have never been tested. They don't know, so we don't know, so we pass along the virus by not knowing. Therefore, I favor testing. When the government called a hear-ing on home-access testing, I wanted to testify.

But at the hearing, I made an even more stunning discov-ery. The primary opposition to home-access testing came from

public clinics and health departments where most AIDS test-
ing is done today. Some feared funding cuts. Others claimed
the urgency of "face-to-face counseling," although none ad-
mitted the truth: few people tested today receive counseling of
any kind. I was shocked to realize that I was arguing against
the good guys, people who every day serve those of us who are
HIV-positive.

I was most baffled by the argument that the government
shouldn't approve home-access testing because some corpora-
tion (read: Johnson & Johnson) might make a profit. I, on the
other hand, hope profits roll in. I want research companies to
believe that discovery of an AIDS cure will earn them billions
of dollars—because that's the day massive research will begin
that could keep me alive.

After I'd testified, the FDA chief caught up to me in a hall-
way. He thanked me and promised "a speedy response and a
quick resolution." So far, no word on FDA approval. Glaciers
move faster than bureaucracies.

In the summer of 1991, after discovering that my husband had
tested positive for the AIDS virus, I learned that I had joined
his ranks. I discovered that, although my children would likely
become AIDS orphans, they were not infected by the virus. And
then came months of deliberation, wrestling with hard questions: Was there purpose in all this? What should I do with my
life? And how should I prepare my children for theirs, if I
should be gone?

Because the virus infects whom it will, several dozen Americans—black and white, gay and straight, old but mostly
young—will become new pilgrims on the road to AIDS between
now and the time you adjourn this evening. We have no fail-safe

means of prevention, so the number of pilgrims increases by the hour. We have no cure, so once a pilgrim starts down this road, there's little question about the final destination.

Since going public with my HIV status in 1992, I've spoken to hundreds of thousands of Americans. In speech after speech, community after community, I've told them—I've asked them, urged them, begged them—to get tested. I've explained how early care can prolong healthy lives. I've pointed to the need to be responsible, so we don't infect those we love. I've encouraged doctors to test more broadly, and communities to embrace more warmly, those who are at risk.

And after two years, I am stunned by the statistics. Less than half of us who are HIV-positive have ever been tested. Without tests, lives are squandered because medical services are skipped; meanwhile, the virus is passed along in ever-increasing numbers to women, adolescents, and children—as well as men.

Testing is terrifying; we dread the results. And the process itself is daunting, especially for women. We're asked to give up anonymity at a time when we feel most vulnerable. Most at-risk women need both transportation and child care if they're to be tested at a clinic; many have neither. The stigma associated with this disease tells us we'll be stamped "dirty women" if we test positive. And data now tells us only 14 percent of those tested ever receive counseling with test results.

On behalf of women, both HIV-positive and HIV-negative, I appeal to you to recommend immediate approval of the Johnson & Johnson home-access HIV testing service.

I can call for testing until I lie down to die, and it will not be enough. My integrity tells me not to defend the status quo, but it does not give me the power to change it. Which distinguishes us—because you do have that power. You can give hundreds of thousands of at-risk people an option. Every survey taken tells us we can double if not triple the number of Americans getting tested, simply by giving them a choice, by letting them test where and when they feel most secure. And you can do that, here, today.

Every week I ask executives to commit their corporations to the battle with AIDS. "Do what you do best," I tell them. In developing the entire system of testing and counseling, Johnson & Johnson—a trusted name in American home health care—is doing exactly what we ask. They are addressing a real marketplace need in such a way that to make a profit they will first make a difference in the epidemic. If they succeed, for every dollar they earn American lives will be lengthened and preserved.

I understand that some, even within the AIDS community, disagree with my perspective. Some defend the existing system, despite its dismal results in both testing and counseling. Others have manufactured hysteria and predicted dire consequences if people are free to choose how and when and where they will be tested.

I would prefer to remember recent history. A generation of hemophiliacs has been erased from our nation because we feared the cost of testing. And critics who oppose giving people options would have us fear their anecdotes today. We would do better to remember history and trust the data.

I was grateful to receive my test results by telephone. It was not the telephone that troubled me, but a doctor who lacked all knowledge about my needs and how I could meet them. Johnson & Johnson has produced a test whose outcome is couched in compassion and referrals to reliable support systems. I cannot help but wonder how much easier my first seven months would have been had their home-access testing service been available to me.

But that is not what I wonder about most. I wonder, more,

whether such an option might have saved my life. "Two out of three people at risk have never been tested"? I can put a name on one of them. His name was Brian. We shared a marriage and two sons and eventually one virus. And now we do not share any of them, because Brian died last year on Father's Day.

Your decision should be made on the basis of the evidence. It shows, by an enormous margin, that the benefits of a home-access option far outweigh the risks.

But your decision, once made, is not merely about statistics. It is about human beings who are dying, one every quarter hour, many of them untested until the autopsy. Your decision, built on hard data, is about marriages and families, about places we go to face our deepest fears, about reasons we hug our children in the night.

It's too late for Brian, and I suppose it's too late for me. But my children are now six and four, and they represent a generation that is not yet lost. Not yet.

For the generation still to come, I urge you, ignore misplaced fears that raise our risks, and trust the facts. Approve home-access testing and give people an option they tell us they will use. Please? Thank you.

WOMEN AND WOUNDED HEALERS

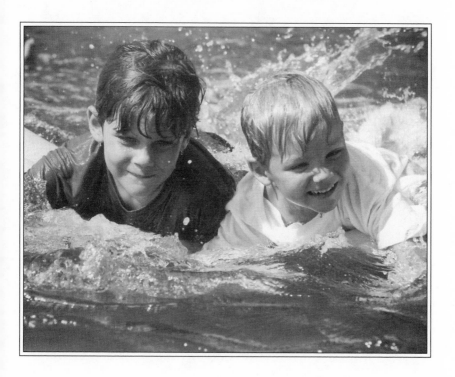

Duke University Continuing Medical Education Conference
Durham, North Carolina
Saturday, June 25, 1994

———

Duke University's Dr. John Bartlett is a good man. He does critical AIDS research. He cares deeply about his colleagues and the people they treat. And he's maintained that improbable balance between a sense of urgency, without which progress cannot be made, and a sense of humor, without which patience disappears before progress occurs. It was he who invited me to address his colleagues at a Duke symposium for physicians.

HIV-positive women, in particular, need supportive physicians. It isn't the fault of the medical community that women are stigmatized; but when stigma finds its way into the medical community, it's especially stubborn and damaging.

Some physicians have learned to steel themselves against pain and loss—and people with AIDS represent both. Medicine cannot save us, and therefore, some medical doctors resent us. They accept us as patients or statistics or clinical trial-participants; they have difficulty accepting us as mothers or lovers or their daughter's nursery-school teacher.

At the same time we see thousands of physicians thoroughly devoted to our well-being. They carry the burdens

shouldered by anyone else, from wayward children to alco-
holic spouses to exhaustion that drains all hope. They are, lit-
erally, wounded healers.

Here was a Saturday evening in June where I could speak
of both groups: women and wounded healers.

A few years ago I only half-joked when I said that I must be
the only HIV-positive Republican. At my children's school and
even often at my doctor's office, it's easy to believe that I'm the
only HIV-positive woman in the neighborhood. Statistics tell
me it isn't true; but I live with people, not statistics. So I was
enormously gratified when I received word of your conference,
calling attention to HIV in women, and I was especially honored at the invitation to join you.

You know, of course, that I am not a physician. I am a woman
living with HIV. By profession, I am an artist; by grace, I'm a
mother; and, by either accident or providence, I'm a pilgrim on
the road to AIDS.

In common with other pilgrims on this road, I take great delight in my company. I have met, as some of you have, people of
enormous courage and dignity who've been infected with this
virus. Among the pilgrims on this road I've found lasting friend-
ships and amazing courage, deep affection and stunning heroism. No clear-thinking pilgrim on the road to AIDS is grateful
for the virus; but it is not uncommon to hear one of us say, "Because of the virus, my life has taken on a new intensity and a
sense of personal meaning that I never knew before."

I did not come this evening to pay tribute to the virus, to give
Pollyannish testimony favoring something that may kill me. The
road to AIDS, no matter how wonderful some of my company
may be, is not the road I would have chosen.

But it's important to me—and, I think, to us—to shift the metaphors we commonly associate with this disease, also in medical communities. I do not get up in the morning, aim some milk at the children's cereal bowl, and say to myself, "I wonder how close to death I am." I am a woman *living* with HIV, grateful to be alive, and grateful when I find partners in the medical community who share my enthusiasm for living.

I live my life as a mother or an artist or a daughter or a friend or even a speaker, but not as a "victim." While your staff may use some form on which I am described as "patient," in the same sense that I have a speaker's form that describes you as "audience," I am not a patient in my day-to-day life, any more than you are an audience. I am what you are: a person.

And it is here that I want to focus my first comment tonight. Because persons with AIDS—among whom I number myself, whether or not I match the CDC definition—and, in particular, women with AIDS, wrestle in some remarkable ways with what psychologists would call "issues of personhood."

Alan Boesak, a black South African leader, once observed that the most convincing proof of apartheid's evil was that it made his children wish they were not black. "When I see them try to wash off the black," he said, "I hear them asking for not merely a different color, but a different identity, and a different father." It was a consequence of evil that Alan could attack, but he could not prevent.

The fact that HIV-positive people in America generally dread having others discover their condition is a result of the same phenomenon: evil. It may be a virus that kills us, but it isn't a virus that drenches us in fear, racks us with guilt, or paralyzes us with shame. People do that, not viruses.

You and I know that the million or more HIV-infected Americans all became infected in exactly the same way: an exchange of bodily fluids. It didn't come from a sneeze or a hug or a shared ice cream cone. It came from an exchange of bodily fluids. Despite this 100-percent certainty, the most frequently asked question I must answer is, "How did you get AIDS?"

Why do you suppose Americans are so obsessive about knowing the individual circumstances of transmission, when we already know with 100-percent certainty how AIDS is transmitted? I suspect it is because our society persists in dividing those with HIV into two camps: those who—to say it indelicately—"got what they deserve," and those who are "innocent victims."

And this is the context in which you come as health-care providers, and I come as a woman living with AIDS, to dinner this evening. Together we face an epidemic of unrivaled historic proportions, which nonetheless must be faced on a one-to-one, person-by-person basis. Although this is clearly a health epidemic, it is one that's discussed by the public at large, and the political establishment in particular, more frequently in moral than in medical terms.

The judgmentalism that brands persons with AIDS is as ugly as the whip used to hurry Jews into boxcars a half century ago. Raised to trust the engine of government in America, I've been stunned to hear language used on the floor of the United States Senate comparing HIV-infected persons with rotten fruit. When I read the fund-raising literature from so-called Christian organizations who view AIDS as an instrument of God, I realize that hatred and meanness are cherished values in some quarters.

This is not some distant, social crisis. This is the defining material for those of us who are HIV-positive. Because it isn't possible to live a human life without hearing human messages about ourselves. That's why Alan Boesak's children tried to wash off the black; that's why HIV-positive people keep quiet about their status. We are merely infected; we're not deaf. We can hear what society says of us.

And what does all this have to do with the patient-doctor relationship? Let me make a few suggestions.

I cannot count the number of times I've been told variations of the following story. An ordinary woman—you, me, your wife, one of our friends—goes to an ordinary physician. The woman is in her twenties or thirties or forties. She's lived an average life, with all the average joys and crises, and a perfectly average number of public triumphs and private intimacies. Having reviewed her life and having scanned the HIV statistics in America, she says to her physician, "Perhaps I could have a test for AIDS." And she hears the response, "You don't need that—you're not that kind of woman."

I mention this first because I want to get it out of the way. I don't imagine you would be here this evening if you were, yourselves, still immersed so deeply in the societal myths that you practice judgmentalism, instead of medicine, in your offices.

But it may be worth a moment of self-examination. The assumptions we make are driven by our beliefs. Whether I am a journalist approaching a story or a priest approaching a sermon or a physician approaching a patient—what I believe shows up in what I do. It may be worth a conversation with a staff person or a colleague.

The gay and hemophiliac communities of America have been ravaged by AIDS. Together, they represent the two moral camps into which we've herded the HIV-positive: those who deserve what they got, and those who are innocent victims. As nearly as I can tell, the virus works exactly the same way in both camps. In both settings, people become sick and die; in both camps, the calls go out for an absent cure; in both camps,

mothers and fathers, brothers and sisters, professional healers
and broken lovers, take turns at the bedside.

But the community you're considering today is one that
America rarely identifies with the AIDS epidemic. It's a community of women: young and old, black and brown and white,
gay and straight, rich and poor, Republican and Democrat. We
are women, living with a disease that our society defines according to its judgments of gay men. We are women, living
largely in silence out of fear that we will lose not only dignity,
but employment; not only insurance, but our children.

I was raised to think of the ideal woman as someone of great
virtue. To be feminine is to be pure. And society tells me that to
have AIDS is to be dirty.

I was trained to think of the ideal woman as someone of great
beauty. To be feminine is to be desirable. And society tells me
that AIDS is repulsive.

When I was a child, nothing could comfort me so completely
as a mother's hug. When I was an adolescent, nothing seemed
as important to me as a young man's embrace. Now I am a
mother, divorced, widowed, and embarrassed to say in public
that I long to be held by someone who wants to hold a woman. I
wonder how many times I've wondered if it is really true that
AIDS has made me, literally, untouchable.

I am grateful for your life and calling as physicians, and I do
not mean to ask that you give up that calling to become psychologists. But I do ask that, in your practice and in your healing, you recognize that women who are, or who may be,
HIV-positive are still women.

We may define our life worth according to some distant sense
of virtue or morality, taught to us by a parish priest or *Father
Knows Best* or an alcoholic mother. It does not matter how we
learned it. What matters is that, if we come to you believing that

to be HIV-positive is to be without virtue, part of your healing must be aimed there, at the belief that we are not worthy.

We may cherish more than you can imagine our roles as mothers or as lovers. We may have defined ourselves too much by our gender, too little by our capacities. It does not matter. What matters is that, if we seek you out, you do not take away from us what gives us meaning.

I understand that health-care professionals must protect themselves both physically and psychologically. You must avoid physical contagion and psychological confusion by using universal precautions in your office and commonsense emotional distance in your life. It all makes sense. I not only understand it, I endorse it for you all.

But can you understand why, as a woman, when I watch the extra gowning and rubber-gloving and whispering behind the screen, I wonder if I am not your partner in the task of healing, but a leper who has wandered in? Can you imagine that some women feel more degraded than helped by their visits to the clinic? Can you see why the power of fear and shame may have a greater impact on our well-being than the drug protocol devised by a stranger at CDC?

The true testimonies of healing are those of people who come into your life broken and leave whole. It is not only, perhaps not even mainly, a matter of blood tests and T-cell counts. My sense of well-being has to do with my sense of self-worth. Without some sense of value, I cannot be whole.

And so I began by saying we are not merely patients, but persons, because I wanted to appeal to you to be not merely technicians, but healers. I wanted to be bold enough this evening to say that, even if I feel to the contrary, I am no less worthy as a person because I have AIDS—and I am no less a woman. I want desperately to believe this, despite what society may say of me. And if you are my caregiver, I would love to see what you can do to convince me that I am right.

Women have traditionally filled the role of caregiver in Western society, and we still do today. One of my colleagues, a man, pointed out a few weeks ago that when we travel together, no one asks him who cares for his children, but people ask me all the time who's caring for mine. It's because we assume that women are the primary caregivers in our homes.

I certainly don't want to fuel false stereotypes of women only as mothers, only as nurses, *only* as helpers. That's neither what I believe nor what has been true in my own life. I'm grateful that men increasingly take on caregiving roles at home and elsewhere, and that women increasingly prove their skills in all settings.

But I mention women as caregivers quite consciously tonight, because when HIV-positive women hear themselves defined by others, they may give up the caregiver role, which is essential both to them and to those around them. If I am defined as a victim, what power do I have to care for others? If I am defined as a patient, what role do I have in healing? If I am defined as an untouchable, a tramp, a moral deviant—you may allow me to retain rights to my children, but would you allow me to take care of yours?

It's critical, I think, for you to encourage HIV-positive women to continue to be caregivers, both for themselves and for others around them. If it is a uniquely feminine experience to have a child nursing at one's breast—and I can assure you that it is—there is also something uniquely feminine that HIV-positive women can bring to their roles as caregivers.

I don't want to exaggerate your responsibility in health care. Many of you are already working inhumane hours that put a unique strain on your personal lives; I sometimes worry about that. Some of you work in conditions of underbudgeted chaos and understaffed crises; I'm familiar with that. And most of you are, frankly, good people. Despite the images sometimes portrayed in the media or elsewhere, you did not pursue careers in caregiving to see how quickly you could buy a mansion or drive a Jaguar. I know.

But I also know, as do you, that physicians and health-care workers occupy unique positions of influence over both public policy and personal well-being. When the AMA speaks, America listens. And when my doctor speaks, I listen.

In matters of public policy, I urge you to be active. Surely I hope you will do what you can, as a health-care professional, to challenge the stigma and discrimination that are still hallmarks of America's AIDS epidemic. Whether in seeking housing for those who are weakened, hospice care for those who are dying, or continued employment for those who are merely infected—those of us on the road to AIDS look to you for support. We recognize that your days and nights are already full of challenge; but we need your voice from time to time.

Some of us are provoked because, even when demographics showed the disease leaving the gay men's community and moving toward other populations, women were rarely involved in necessary studies. We know less today about the course of HIV in women than in men because research has been influenced by prejudice and politics. We know that, for physiological reasons, women are uniquely susceptible to the virus. And all these factors are reasons why we value your public voice, as representatives of the medical community, when matters of public policy are up for grabs.

You do a great deal, each of you, in your healing profession. But if you can do more to combat ignorance and encourage compassion, I would be most grateful to you.

It was Norman Cousins who taught us that "the opposite of love is not hate. It's indifference." It's a worthy slogan to remember when we are taking on public policy.

But it may have even greater value if we could remember it not only in public, but also in private, in our personal and day-to-day exchanges with our families and our friends and our colleagues.

It would be irresponsible of me not to at least mention that some of you have probably been at risk for HIV and have not been tested. You have all the knowledge in the world about risk factors, and about your own lives. But you don't want to know. If you love yourself, or if you love someone else, you cannot be indifferent. Get tested.

Most of you have families in which it's easy to assume that someone else will do the teaching; after all, look at your hours and your dedication to medicine. How can anyone expect you to do more? I could tell you a story about going with my doctor to his daughter's school to speak, and what my doctor learned about his daughter in that setting. I am grateful you are health-care professionals. In my view, your knowledge equips you to do more in your families—it does not exempt you.

But if I could urge a single proposal here this evening, it would be that you model love for one another.

I am grateful for scientific advances and laboratory discoveries. God knows, I pray for more because I pray for a cure. But when we turn from the matter of scientific discovery to the practice of health-care delivery, I take a new and lively interest in how you relate to one another.

When I enter a clinic where doctors never speak to one another, where nurses are treated as necessary evils and office staff are regarded as cost centers, I realize that I've come to a place of business. But I do not believe I have come to a place of healing. If it is all a matter of business, then I am only worth the insurance card I present—and if I have no card, I have no worth. I suspect, though I may be wrong, that not many of you here tonight are among those for whom health care is merely a matter of business.

What I suspect is that I have here an audience of health-care professionals who worry about keeping enough distance from their professions to save their marriages, enough time in their weeks to prove that they can still be a lover or a parent or a friend. I do not really suspect you of being cold entrepreneurs. I imagine that you are less in danger of treating me as a number than in danger of crying hard when someone you care about dies. I imagine that you are frustrated with the paperwork and politics of health care, and that there is less indifference in this room than pain.

I imagine that some of you have slammed your fists into walls when the child died, and others have driven home more than once saying you'll never go back again, never become involved again, never, never, never hurt again. And then you got up the next day and you went back to it: the chaos, the uncertainty, the confusion, and the pain. Not because you wanted to be wealthy, but because you wanted to be true to yourself.

I think I understand this. I've given up on giving speeches so often, it would make your head swim. I've said to myself, I will never again be naked about the shame of this disease in front of another audience, I will never again be vulnerable. I'm going to take my children and run and hide.

So here we are together, wounded healers and a weary speaker. Where do we go, what do we do?

I have a suggestion. Rather than hiding behind the thin veil of professionalism, why don't we simply admit to one another that we, too, are in pain, we, too, are frightened, and we, too, need to be lifted up when we are weary and comforted when we are broken? Professionalism has its place, but denial is suicidal and indifference kills those around us.

Not only HIV-positive women, but all those who come to you, want to be cared for. And so do you. You want me to know, when I come into your office, that I have what you cannot fix. You want me not to blame you for the cancer that will find me, for the wasting that will weaken me, for the fear in my children's eyes when they finally realize what all this means. In your efforts to heal me, you may well be heroic; but in the quiet moments when you've lost me, you are utterly and unmistakably human.

Where do we go? What do we do? We might try going to each other. We might try embracing one another. Already we are people. But if we are to heal or be healed, we will need to become partners. Neither you nor I would partner with someone who judges us morally inferior and professionally distasteful. But I would welcome and celebrate and sing praises for those who set aside their professional veneer and attitudes of indifference to embrace me. There is a power in such moments that washes over both the healer and those seeking healing.

I wish you a moment of reflection this evening, a time of laughter with one another, and tomorrow, a day of renewed affection. And, until the day we hold healing in our hands together, I offer you this ancient prayer: grace to you, and peace.

UNTIL
THERE'S A CURE

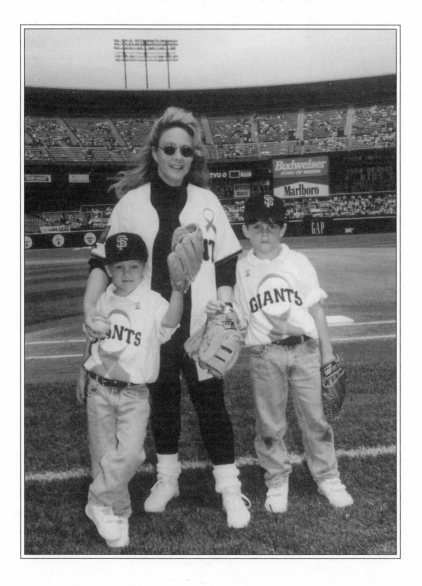

San Francisco Giants "Until There's a Cure Day"
Candlestick Park
San Francisco, California
Sunday, July 31, 1994

———

The San Francisco Giants, ardently supported by owner Peter McGowan, became the first major professional sports franchise to sponsor a day to benefit AIDS causes. They sold out Candlestick Park, raised funds for research and care, and set a model for others.

Part of the pregame ceremony was the formation by hundreds of red-shirted and red-capped people, most HIV-positive, of a massive, human AIDS awareness ribbon in center field. After I'd spoken, several members of the Giants team were to symbolize solidarity by walking out to join them.

But instead of a token player or two, all the Giants headed for center field. As they left the infield, Barry Bonds waved to the Colorado Rockies dugout inviting them to join—and they did, every one of them. As music filled the stadium, baseball heroes hugged HIV-infected men and women, and fifty-three thousand fans roared approval in a standing, tear-soaked ovation.

Of all the wonderful things about that day, none was more

wonderful than this: the Giants, for one whole day, made it okay
to have AIDS. The sickness weakens you and the dying nearly
breaks you. But for one warm, magical day in the stadium by
the bay, no one with AIDS was made to feel unworthy.

On behalf of the more than one million Americans infected with AIDS, I am here to salute the San Francisco Giants.

While parents across the nation deny the epidemic that stalks their children, Dusty Baker looks at his daughter, Natosha, and says, "We must act." Today, a million of us who are pilgrims on the road to AIDS know Dusty Baker is a hero.

Long before he took the hand of my son Max, Rod Beck began caring for children with AIDS—not before the camera, but with his wife, Stacey, in the quiet of their home. Today, more than a million of us want Rod and Stacey Beck to know: they are heroes along the road to AIDS.

Young and gifted, able to join any cause, Royce Clayton did not fear being identified with AIDS. A remarkable player, he's a more remarkable man hugging my son Zack. A million pilgrims on the road to AIDS will not need to sew his name into the Quilt to remember it. We know heroes when we see them.

For a decade and a half, America at large has said that AIDS is not our problem, not our disease. It belongs to "your" community or "their" community or no community at all, but it does not belong to us. Fever by night and cancer by day—if it is AIDS, it is not ours. We have clung to our denial, passing judgment on those the virus finds, imagining that it belongs to those less worthy, less moral, less righteous, than ourselves. We have cherished our prejudices, loved our stigma, and forgotten that God makes some pilgrims strong so they can carry the weak.

Today, the San Francisco Giants demonstrate that AIDS is as

all-American as Abner Doubleday's sport. No longer can we deny that this epidemic is all of ours. No longer must men and women and children hide in fear and shame as they grow weak and die. Because good men in San Francisco are not only baseball's Giants, but moral giants as well.

For fifteen years, some here today have fought to replace the shroud of stigma with a quilt of justice; today, they have won. Let the word go out that those not yet infected have joined the pilgrim band. Those not HIV-positive will the take the hand of those who are. They will speak to us of courage. They will comfort us as we grow weak. They will burn the midnight oil to unlock the secret that will save our lives, until there's a cure.

For years the red ribbon has represented awareness and hope. Today, we see athletes and heroes not only wearing the ribbon, but joining as part of it. Today, men of honor join us on the road to AIDS—not because they are infected by the virus, but because they are compassionate.

Until there's a cure, pilgrims on the road to AIDS will grow weary. We fear the end of this road. We grow frightened. We see our children, and we grow sad.

But today, we see strong hands reaching out to hold my children. We see the confidence of a six-year-old embraced by a pitcher, and the grace that flows from a shortstop's hug. The Quilt is for our memory, the ribbon for our hope; but we, who are alive today, we are for one another.

So let the word go out, from Candlestick Park, that today we are all pilgrims on the road to AIDS. Infected and uninfected, weak and strong. Let those who would be heroes reach down to lift a child and reach out to comfort the dying. And let those who are giants among us carry those too weak to carry on.

Until there's a cure, let there be love.

LISTENING
FOR GOD'S ECHO

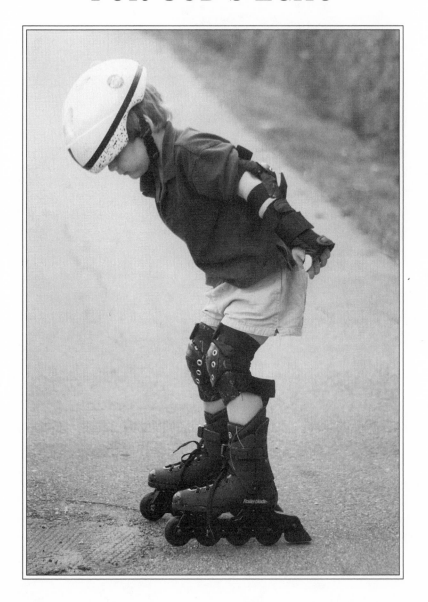

Toms River Presbyterian Church
Toms River, New Jersey
September 25, 1994
[Delivered Sunday, December 4, 1994]

———

Toms River Presbyterian Church, nestled in the New Jersey countryside not far from the Atlantic, an hour south of New York City, had a pastor—the Reverend Dr. Blair Monie—who, with his wife, Cyndy, had read Sleep with the Angels, *my first anthology of speeches and photographs. They responded by writing a letter, inviting a sermon.*

I'd struggled through several months of borderline depression. Jim and I had spent long hours in conversation. And his first draft of the sermon had captured exactly what I wanted to say. I was eager to preach again.

Then came the flu. Tuesday I was down, protesting that I was not out. Wednesday was worse; I couldn't talk at all. Thursday we were treating a virus and maybe a sinus infection; I was on antibiotics, feeling rotten. By Friday we did what we'd never done before: canceled an appearance.

Starting the following Tuesday, each day's mail—for weeks—brought cards from Toms River containing gifts for the Family AIDS Network and promising prayer for my recov-

ery. It was not as I had planned it. But I am not certain that, in the larger scheme of things, it wasn't planned.

THE OLD TESTAMENT READING: I KINGS 19: 4, 11–15

But [Elijah] went a day's journey into the wilderness and came and sat down under a solitary broom tree. He asked that he might die: "It is enough; now, O Lord, take away my life. . . ." [And the Voice] said, "Go out and stand on the mountain before the Lord, for the Lord is about to pass by."

Now there was a great wind, so strong that it was splitting mountains and breaking rocks in pieces before the Lord, but the Lord was not in the wind; and after the wind an earthquake, but the Lord was not in the earthquake; and after the earthquake a fire, but the Lord was not in the fire; and after the fire a sound of sheer silence.

When Elijah heard it, he wrapped his face in his mantle and went out and stood at the entrance of the cave. Then there came a voice to him that said, "What are you doing here, Elijah?"

He answered, "I have been very zealous for the Lord, the God of hosts; for the Israelites have forsaken your covenant, thrown down your altars, and killed your prophets with the sword. I alone am left, and they are seeking my life, to take it away."

Then the Lord said to him, "Go, return on your way."

THE NEW TESTAMENT READING: JAMES 5: 13–18

Are there any among you suffering? They should pray. Are any cheerful? They should sing songs of praise. Are any among you sick? They should call for the elders of the church and have them pray over them, anointing them with oil in the name of the Lord. The prayer of faith will save the sick, and the Lord will raise them up; and anyone who has committed sins will be forgiven. Therefore, confess your sins to one another and pray for one another, so that you may be healed.

The prayer of the righteous is powerful and effective. Elijah was a human being like us, and he prayed fervently that it might not rain, and for three years and six months it did not rain on the earth. Then he prayed again, and the heaven gave rain and the earth yielded its harvest.

I have two confessions with which to begin. The first is that, before September, I'd never heard of Toms River, New Jersey. After receiving so much mail from you, and looking forward eagerly to meeting you this morning, I'll never again forget either your location or your kindness.

The second confession is harder: I had an ecumenical childhood. I was raised in a Jewish home and attended a school in the Episcopalian tradition. But the only place I'd ever heard of Presbyterians was in a piece by one of my favorite authors, Mark Twain. His short story "A Dog's Tale" was written in the voice of a puppy. I loved that story, but I was seriously misled by it. Because it opens with this sentence: "My father was a St. Bernard and my mother was a collie; but I am a Presbyterian."

I blame Twain for the fact that I was seventeen before I could distinguish a Presbyterian from a wolfhound.

Now that I'm here with you, I see the difference. Nearly all of you are human. I'm encouraged by this, because it means we have something in common with a hero of the faith. "Elijah was a human being like us," according to our New Testament lesson.

If we think of the Bible as a book about superhumans, we'll miss the point of this morning's story. Because it's all about being just, plain human.

Elijah *is* extraordinary. He calls up droughts and then prays them to an end. When he's thirsty, God leads him to a cooling stream; when he's hungry, God fills a widow's cupboard so she can feed him. He prays, and God sends fire; he prays again, and a child comes back from the dead. It's no wonder that James, when he wrote the letter from which we read this morning, felt the need to remind his readers that Elijah was just "a human being like us."

The Old Testament passage this morning proves Elijah's humanness. Hard times have come. He's frightened, discouraged, tired. He's cowering under a bush where he wants to die. The man we meet isn't remembering his miracles; he's depressed and working on suicide. And things don't improve when he slogs his way up the mountain for a promised visit by God. In fact, life becomes more of an ordeal.

Elijah knew that God had visited Israel before in wind and in earthquakes and in fire. But here, on the mountain, with the wind blasting rocks around Elijah's head, "the Lord was not in the wind." Something was wrong.

Then came earthquakes, but "the Lord was not in the earthquake." Something was terribly wrong.

Jagged spears of lightning split the darkened sky, but "the Lord was not in the fire." Elijah—depressed, suicidal—was on the mountain alone; no God.

Then came the "sound of sheer silence," and a Voice—like the voice of a father or mother as they lift a frightened child out of the darkness and into their bed: "What's the matter, Max?" "What do you need, Zack?"—"What are you doing here, Elijah?"

It's a remarkable story about a very human man.

Three years ago I made a discovery about my own humanness. First a man who'd been my husband called, and then a doctor I hardly knew called, and then I knew that I had contracted the virus that causes AIDS. It was earthquakelike news, breaking everything delicate in my life. Days before my then four- and two-year-old sons were sunshine children building backyard kingdoms; now I saw them playing only in shadows. I didn't know how I would help them through their father's death; and what would I tell them of my own?

But families rally. Friends turn into heroes. Self-pity gives way to responsibility as we realize that ours is a story shared by a million or more Americans who are today pilgrims on the road to AIDS. To be HIV-positive is not such an unusual thing anymore.

I've occasionally joked that I knew just what Elijah meant when he said that "I and only I am left," because I felt like the only HIV-positive Republican in America. But the fact is, if there's value in my life story, it isn't that something is unusual but that my life is ordinary. Including some recent months that have been especially hard. I've had the feeling that God was absent from me, and I think it's important to talk about it for a moment.

My life since childhood has been busy and full. After becoming a mother, I'd always welcomed the quiet time after my sons were asleep. But somewhere this past spring I realized I didn't welcome these times at all. I felt my mood begin to swing. Alone time in the evening became grinding, grief-filled, lonesome times that lasted through the night and left me drained and limp in the morning.

Last June I told a gala dinner audience that I was weary of giving speeches, that I'd lost all hope of changing attitudes, that I saw no reason to keep fighting denial and stigma and discrimination. Most of them, I suppose, thought it was rhetorical flourish; but it wasn't. It was an honest admission. I'd given up believing that what I said or did would matter—or that I would. If I was to have purpose, life needed meaning—and I couldn't find any. If I was to be called, Someone needed to call me—and I couldn't hear anyone. Too tired to work during the day, too anxious to sleep at night, when I cried out for God, begging him to make a house call, I heard only the sound of sheer silence.

Shall I just say it? I could not take my life because of my sons. And I did not want my life because it—because I—did not matter.

The Bible describes Elijah as a solitary man, the only one standing for God, the last great hero—that is, until just after the passage we read this morning. Elijah came down the mountain never to be alone again. God sent him a companion in the person of Elisha, who ultimately carried on his work. Elisha was not God, but he was a mirror of God's companionship, showing Elijah that he was not really alone. Elisha was not God's voice, but he was God's echo: in him, Elijah could hear the sound of God at work.

Elijah came down the mountain, and I've come out of the valley, having heard the echo of God's footsteps, the whisper of a still, small voice. And the message that has stayed with me is all about comfort for those who want to listen.

It's a comfort to know that *feeling* God's absence doesn't *make* God absent. It's like the experience of having someone you love not come home on time. You notice a distant siren. You think you hear screaming tires and see shattered glass; you watch the sad surgeon come slowly down the hallway of your imagination. You feel their loss so deeply that when they come through the door for dinner, you want to kill them for putting you through such terror.

Fearing it, feeling it, didn't make it real; the same is true of missing God. Feeling his absence does not make him absent.

But one of the great dangers of such times is that we lose perspective, not only on ourselves but also on God.

I was with Brian, my children's father, when he died. Brian was not sure what was happening in the next life; his comfort level was sometimes low. There were days when we were both washed with agony and forgiveness and good-byes. It was not a time I want to revisit, really.

But I remembered it and understood it differently a month ago when a friend told me of C. S. Lewis. Lewis, a great believer, helped his wife through an agonizing death from cancer. In the hours after her death, he wrote:

> Not that I am . . . in much danger of ceasing to
> believe in God. The danger is of coming to
> believe such dreadful things about him. The
> conclusion I dread is not 'So there's no God after
> all,' but 'So this is what God is really like. . . .'

As I wrestled with the grief of losing not only my husband, Brian, but also Arthur and Jeffrey and Pedro and Elizabeth and, oh, so many others—and my sense that, when I saw them going, I was looking in a mirror—my sense of loss had made me question, perhaps for the first time in my life, what God is really like. It's a hard question for the million or so pilgrims on the road to AIDS, and those who love us.

One reason it's hard is that not everyone has told the truth. We've heard self-righteous bigots pound their pulpits, raising tempers and raising money with brutalities. They've declared that AIDS is God's punishing instrument of justice. They've succeeded in making some who know they're sick believe that they're also damned. And they've kept aging parents from telling the truth about their children's wasting illness, for fear that they, too, will be judged evil.

When we cannot feel God's presence, when we are frightened or depressed, we may not know how to answer such charges. But I'm feeling well now, and I know precisely what I would say. I'd tell such spiritual impostors that theirs is a venerable tradition of hatred, but it is no gospel. A century ago their ancestors lit the burning crosses that warmed slowly twisting bodies of lynched black men. A half century ago their fathers turned away from the Holocaust to mutter that the Jews had it coming. Its not tradition they lack, but truth. They are windows on hell, not mirrors of God. And someone should say so.

But there's another religious extreme that may, in the long run, be even more damaging: people filled with sympathy who never move beyond their momentary feelings. They hear a speech, they read a book; "We'll do all we can," they say. And they do nothing. Peter Marshall described them as "all dressed up for deep-sea diving, marching off bravely to pull plugs out of bathtubs." Exactly. They want to be seen as heroes, without the bother of heroism. They want to be thought charitable without getting too close to the sick or hungry. They want to be as religiously correct as possible with as little inconvenience as necessary. If others contributed substantially to my long hours of doubt, these were the primary donors.

From the perspective of the AIDS community, these are more dangerous than the judgmental fanatic, because it's hard to understand why good people would do nothing in the face of so many deaths.

If in God's name we promise to act, but don't, what are others to believe? And if I'm genuinely persuaded that the people of God do not care, how do I answer the obvious question: "So this is what God is really like?"

Tears distort our vision and cloud our view. Grief and depression make us wonder where God has gone. It's unavoidable. But what's even more unforgettable is this: the moment of comfort—that slow, sweet, healing time when relieving comfort rolls in. One day the shadow is less black. One night the comforter is cuddly, and you snuggle in. One morning you wake and realize that you want to see the children and taste the day's first cup of coffee; you wonder what the day will bring. Because God has finally paid the house call.

For Elijah, there was Elisha—a man who echoed God's grace when most Elijah could not hear it on his own. What about us? What about me, what about you—do you know where we can hear the echo of God's footsteps in the course of our busy lives, in the context of a deadly epidemic, in the closing days of this millennium?

I've heard God's soft echo in rooms of dying men whose parents have become their caregivers. I've held the hand of a man who came out of a coma to bless me. His family had hardly been able to accept him as gay; surely, they could not accept him as dying. His father, a big-city cop for three decades, had seen everything there was to see. Until that final night, when he walked slowly to his son's bed, bent over his child, and began to pray. I saw that night a hardened man so softened by grace that I could not doubt the power of God. I heard a gentle murmur of hope, enough to make me believe again.

In hospices and hospital rooms, friends' apartments and family mansions, the echo of God's love whispers courage to those who are sick and comfort to those who are dying. Ask a nurse from an AIDS ward where she finds strength to go back again, and you may be surprised to hear her speak of God. Ask a doctor who has nothing scientific left with which to fight the virus, "How do you do it? How do you lose so many that you love?" Better yet, come in yourself. Give up your fear of those who suffer, your terror at the prospect of seeing death up close. Become a caregiver, and listen to what you hear in the silence.

My children are now seven and five. We've stumbled through their father's death together, and like most of you, we stumble

through life. Some days are cheerful songs and others are funeral dirges as we live out the contrasts of the childhood song:

> Ring around the rosies, pocket full of posies
> Ashes! Ashes! We all fall down. . . .

An extraordinary grief accompanies the thought that one's
children may too soon be orphans. But so does a sense of extraordinary humanness. We are born, we live, we serve a little
while, we die. Dust to dust, ashes to ashes . . . we all fall down.

And meanwhile, some of you are strong and gifted, full of grace
and truth. I know it personally because I've read your letters to
me. You are God's gift to me and to this congregation, to your home
and to your community. When you see children who are susceptible to illness because of ignorance or poverty; women who are
vulnerable because they cannot protect themselves; men and
women who are sick and infected because they did not believe
they were at risk—what a wonderful occasion God has given you
to prove just who you are: strong, gifted, full of grace and truth.
It's an opportunity to prove that you are not content merely to say
something nice; you can do something stunningly good.

Some of you have, like me, wrestled for a sign of God's presence in your life. You have been in the valley of depression. You
have wrestled with the darkest fears. I have this one suggestion
for you: stop wrestling. Tell the truth about your terror to someone you trust, then sit quietly together some night, listening to the
silence. You may discover that you don't really need desperately
to grab hold of God. Because He's holding you gently in His hand.
When you see that grace, you will feel His peace.

Which is why, today, this is not only my prayer for you; it is
also my promise: grace to you, and peace.

TAKING
HOLD OF INTEGRITY

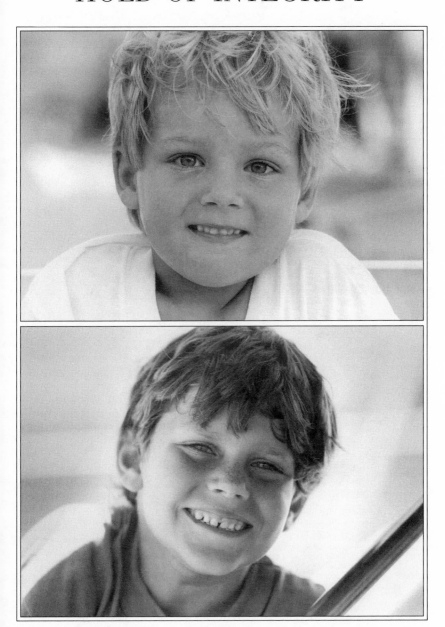

AIDS Task Force of Alabama Annual Awards Dinner
Montgomery, Alabama
Thursday, October 6, 1994

———

Billy Cox came out of his hospital bed in Birmingham, Alabama, to bring me a hug in Montgomery.

I'd first met him a year earlier at the University of Alabama at Birmingham where I was visiting Michael Saag, a recognized AIDS researcher, a wonderful physician, and my cousin. Michael wanted me to meet Billy, to see his spunk and spirit. "Billy's the boxer in the ring," Michael once observed. "The doctors and nurses and medical staff, we're just the trainers in his corner. His friends and family are his fans, cheering him on."

Now, a year later, I'd come to Montgomery to speak about community, about bridging gaps that divide us, about enabling us to live and die together. But what I said was not as eloquent as the events that soon played out in the life of Boxer Billy and Cousin Michael.

Six weeks after he'd brought his hug to Montgomery— seven years, four months, and three days after testing positive for the AIDS virus—Billy Cox died. November 23, 1994.

On Billy's last day, Michael Saag was leaving town for a few days and stopped in just to say good-bye. When he heard

*Billy's labored breathing, he called the family together and
told them the end was near. And then—as nurses and old
friends and Billy's family crowded into the room, forming a
remarkable community bound only by love for the boxer—
Michael rested his head on Billy's chest and, unashamed before the crowd, sobbed, "I'm sorry, I'm sorry."*

*Science has limits. Even community has bounds. But no
one will ever know what love might do.*

Of all the communities in America, none is more familiar with
statistics than the AIDS community. If we had a group portrait,
ours might be a paint-by-numbers image. Whatever else we
know, we always know the grim numbers.

We know rates of death, now momentarily slowed because
the pace of infection momentarily slowed ten years ago as
America's gay and hemophiliac communities responded to the
first wave. We know these rates will accelerate again in about
two years. And we know about how many members of Congress
vote as if they care.

We know the AIDS virus is spreading most rapidly among
adolescents and women today. We know that death follows infection by roughly a decade, so we're now discovering where
the virus traveled one year before President Reagan first said
the word *AIDS* in public. And we know that, while we enjoy
each other's company this evening, a dozen of our colleagues
will die.

Some of us know numbers that suggest not only the size of
this community, but even the length of our life. Our best friend
whispers, "How are your numbers?"; someone we love calls to
say, "My numbers went under one hundred . . . "; we know
these numbers too well.

Numbers may define size or progression, but they do not define character. And I'm hopeful this evening that you might join me in working on character—specifically, the character of an enduring community in which all members are encouraged to live with dignity and die with courage. I'm here to ask that you help me build an AIDS community that is worthy of our children.

We know, of course, that we cannot have integrity alone. The first meaning of the word *integrity* isn't honesty; it's wholeness or completeness. And we cannot be whole, we are not complete, by ourselves. It's in our caregiving and caretaking, our loving and our being loved—which is to say, in our life with others— that we define ourselves and our characters.

The same is true of the AIDS community. A million or two of us are pilgrims on the road to AIDS; we were drafted into this struggle. But millions of others, including most of you, enlisted. Some of you came because of your profession: you saw an opportunity, and you took it. Some of you came because of your values: you saw a need, and you met it. And many first came because you loved one certain pilgrim: you came to hold his hand or make her smile. And when you needed to let go of them, you stayed. Whatever brought you into the AIDS community, I'm grateful you are here with me.

Since we're here, together, I have an idea: let's build a community so sturdy that mean men and thoughtless women can do it no damage. Let's create a classroom for compassion, where children spend their days learning lessons not of cruelty but of courage, not of bias but of grace. Let's create a community that's worthy of the name.

I know we need such a community because I have two children, ages six and four. Their understanding is going to be shaped by their community, including their understanding of what happened first to their father and then to their mother.

And I know that we can build such a community because, face-to-face with life and death, people do heroic things—and the AIDS community has thousands of stories to prove such heroism.

Still, we have a long way to go if we're to create an AIDS community that's fully vested with integrity and decorated with hope. And if I were to propose a first step, it would be this: we need to reshape our understanding of the AIDS community itself.

We assumed from the beginning that the struggle with AIDS would be acute, not chronic; that our scientists would go into their laboratories one day and come out the next bearing a cure, perhaps a preventative. Grassroots and national organizations alike rose up to fight a short fight, to win a quick victory, to score a few points and go home. And much of the early leadership came from those who were, themselves, infected.

But now we know that this is not going to be a brief battle with a glorious ending. We're in a long and bloody crusade. Hundreds of thousands have already fallen, millions more are marked, and there's no end in sight.

To build an AIDS community with integrity, a place my children and yours can finish their growing years, we need to build a community that will endure.

If you think this is some vague abstraction, especially those of you who are HIV-negative, think again. Because those of us who are infected are, truly, pilgrims on the road to AIDS. We're passing through the community and can give it leadership or service for only a little while. In those moments when we hold our children or cradle our lovers, we might trade anything to stay a little longer. But we cannot. And we will not. And we know that now.

Arthur Ashe left a sterling legacy; but he's not able to lead the cause tonight. Ryan White is memorialized in legislation, but will not walk the halls of Congress tomorrow. There are limits to the leadership that can be provided by those of us who are infected. One limit is illness; another is death. And we know that now.

Therefore, to build an AIDS community with staying power, we must build on leadership from those who are uninfected as well as those who are infected. We need institutions that do not weaken when founders grow weak and do not perish when founders must take their leave. We need the passion of those who are infected and the strength of those who are not. The AIDS community needs partnerships from here on out. We need *un*infected people making their life commitment to this community. Or the community itself will, like many within in it, waste and perish.

And if we're to revitalize the AIDS community, we need—in the second place—to be aggressive in defining and defending the community's moral position.

Whole pockets of this nation still believe AIDS is a gay disease. It betrays an ignorance that condemns our national claims to education. That such ignorance is alive and well in 1994 is stunning.

What's worse, in some of these pockets there's great rejoicing that the disease is reducing the number of gay men in America. They think of others, like me, as "innocent victims," but hold that gay men deserve their fate. When this brutality finds its way into houses of worship, the Creator God is re-created by narrow-minded little men in their own ugly image. And then we are fighting not only stereotypes but outright evil.

I want to say, unambiguously, that it's time for our community to stand up to moral thugs and speak a word on behalf of compassion and grace. We've had far too much of bashful silence and far too little of vigorous truth. In meetings of school boards and county boards; in assemblies of church and state; at family reunions and factory dinners—we need to shame bigots who delight in prejudice and challenge cowards who don't dare tell the children the truth. Candidates who lack the decency to embrace the sick, care for the dying, and protect the orphan lack the basic integrity that earns our vote.

A community is defined in part by what it says. But we've been so silent as a community that America at large can hardly imagine we number in the millions, or that we have anything important to say.

A community is defined in part by what it does. But what moral courage do we show if—a decade and a half into the epidemic—we dare not stand up to be counted?

To become a community that endures, we need to embrace a message loaded with strong values—and then we must speak that message loudly and model that image boldly. Science does not promise us hope today. Unless the community is willing to fight for right values, neither we nor our children will find any hope at all.

Third, we need to remember that communities are created; they do not just "happen." They are rooted in a sense of shared values and shared interests. They are nurtured by an understanding of their history and destiny. But we must plant them, and we must tend them.

John Gardner, adviser to Presidents Kennedy, Johnson, Carter, and Reagan—and now a professor at Stanford University—observed that communities need "ceremonies and celebrations that provide bonding experiences." He noted that most of us aren't even aware of how important these rituals are.

"For many of my university colleagues," said Gardner, "the whole idea of engaging in ritual celebration seems somehow corny. But then commencement time comes and we all put on medieval robes and march to eighteenth-century music and do a great job of celebrating our own tradition."

In a small German village, not long after the Second World War, a new rabbi was assigned to a newly rebuilt temple. During his first days there, he noticed that each evening around dusk, a workman rode up on his bike, went briefly into the temple, and then came out and rode away. He was tall, broadshouldered, blond-haired, and blue-eyed—by every appearance not a Jew.

One day, curious, the rabbi listened at the temple door during the man's brief visit. And what he heard, in flawless Hebrew, were the words of Judaism's most sacred text, the ancient Shema: *"Shema, Isroel, Adonoi, Eloheanu, Adonoi Ehad"*— "Hear, O Israel, the Lord our God, the Lord is One."

As the workman left the temple, the rabbi was waiting, and asked, "Are you Jewish?"

"No." For the first time, the man turned his face toward the rabbi. It was an old face on a young German, and he knew the rabbi's question. "I was the one who sealed the doors of the gas chambers. The last thing I heard each time was, *"Shema, Isroel, Adonoi, Eloheanu . . ."*

Ritual is important to shaping a community. It defines us at critical moments; it lends us language when other words fail. The Fourth of July and Thanksgiving provide ritual moments that tell us that "we, the people," are American. Stories kept and told by the slaves became the ritual that eventually gave rise to a spirit of strength and dignity in a community that had known only captivity and servitude. Adult children who've long since left the faith of their fathers can still hear their fathers' voices in prayer. We are defined and our communities are affirmed by ritual celebrations.

It's true of the AIDS community, too. AIDS walks first conceived to raise funds now raise awareness as well—showing our neighbors that we know not only how to lobby, but how to laugh; that we have strength not only to march in protest but also to walk in celebration. World AIDS Day needs to be observed. So do prayer vigils in which we call out names of those who've gone before us. We light candles to tell loved ones that we have not forgotten. And we go quietly to our national memorial, the NAMES Project Quilt, to walk amid our memories, grieve promises cut short a day or two ago, and promise our children a better tomorrow.

In Alabama as elsewhere, we must not assume our community; we must build it. We must break down whatever barriers exist between black and white, gay and straight, infected and uninfected—especially in the AIDS community, these differences are mere trifles. When you are straight and white and dying, you welcome having your fevered brow cooled by a black hand, your sores tended by a gay nurse, your family comforted by an uninfected chaplain. A community divided by any stigma cannot call others to give up prejudice. And a community divided will not endure.

It's in community—glorious, affirming community—that we learn to laugh at ourselves, sing of our triumphs, and be lifted up when we fall down. It's in community with others that we receive the joy needed to carry on. Which is one of the reasons we gather tonight: to celebrate achievement, to laugh, to cry, to love.

These are my calls to you, my brothers and sisters in the AIDS community of Alabama: recognize that the AIDS community is engaged in a long-term struggle requiring leadership that partners the infected and the uninfected; take the truth to war against wrong values and mean judgments; and remember that communities are created—they do not just "happen."

And with those calls, this one plea: do not give up and do not give in. Don't be intimidated by death, seduced by professionalism, or tempted to think of defeat. If you feel yourself sinking, call out; someone in the community will rescue you.

America has an enormous capacity to deny the reality of death. We tell endless stories of beginnings and childhood. We celebrate birthdays with cards and cakes and other rituals that do much for humor and little for dignity. We cannot get enough of talking about birth and everything that's happened since. And if you want to stop a cocktail party conversation, raise your voice just a little and say, "Death."

The AIDS community cannot deny death; it lacerates every banner we hang and decorates with grief every memorial we create. It is part of us, a defining characteristic that sets us apart from most American communities. It is a critical component of who we are. And by accepting the fact that death lives among us, more as a full-time resident than an occasional tourist, we gain a strength that is unmatched in most Western communities.

I'd never seen death so close until Brian asked me to be with him at the end. We'd loved each other and married; we'd fought and divorced. Now we shared two sons and one virus and a desire not to be alone at the end.

It was a visiting nurse who explained to me about blue fingernails and stiffening hands. But no one could explain to me the meaning of a final "I love you" that said that forgiveness had taken the place of anger. No one could prepare me to hear him whisper, "Say good-bye to the boys—I miss them already." No one could explain how to say, "It's all right, Brian, you can let go now. It's enough. You don't need to fight anymore." But we don't need to explain this much in the AIDS community, because so many of us have been there.

To deny the potency of death is to cheat the AIDS community

of one of its most defining elements: tangible, throbbing grief. But it is also to steal from us what makes us strong. Because, having faced death up close and personal, we've defeated what other communities can only deny.

Take the measure of death, and you'll no longer fear foolish politicians or cowardly preachers. Take the measure of death, and you'll understand something about values for life: the importance of truthfulness in our relationships, the uselessness of things, the joy of Billy Cox being here to hug me, and the sweetness of a child's sleepy kiss.

Don't be intimidated by death; don't give in to America's denial. And those of you who've volunteered for this duty—who are here not because you are infected but because you care—don't be seduced by too much professionalism.

Caregivers are the heroes in this struggle. It is all of you, not just a few award winners, who must be honored this evening. But I want to warn you: You've been taught as a nurse to keep your distance from the patients, lest you risk identification with them. You've been taught as a social worker or as a volunteer not to take on the burdens of your clients, lest you risk confusion with them. You've been encouraged as a pastor to maintain discreet distance; as an administrator not to get bogged down in the details of individual lives.

I want you to care for yourselves and your families. I want you not to burn out. Protect yourselves with common sense.

But you can't maintain professional distance, to keep from feeling the terrible losses, and still bring me comfort. You can't pull back from the stinging grief that accompanies each death or stave off the fear that haunts us through the night and still say you love me.

If you will care for us, then care. Don't hide. Don't run. Don't quit. Care. That means, in other words: Risk. Love. Hurt. Embrace. Hope. Laugh. And, fervently, pray.

Instead of workshops on burnout, try this ancient creed: "Weep with those who mourn, and laugh with those who rejoice." Instead of applauding me safely, try hugging me tightly. Instead of retreating from the pain, embrace it—*and then share it*—and you will find that when you let the community bear it with you, it will not break you. If you will participate in community, you will discover pools of cooling comfort and streams flowing with joy.

And do not, *do* not, do *not* believe that we will be defeated by this virus.

It was Herb Daniel, the great Brazilian poet claimed by AIDS in 1992, who wrote: "I hope that one day, when death finally comes, by chance or by any infection caused by the virus, nobody says that I was defeated by AIDS. I have succeeded in living with AIDS. AIDS has not defeated me."

Precisely. AIDS has no more power to defeat us than the virus that causes the common cold. And it is the sacred purpose of the AIDS community—infected and uninfected, strong and weak—to affirm this truth over and over and over again.

We come, as a community, to those who lead our corporations and our civic agencies, and we demand justice and compassion—not because some of us are dying, but because all of us are living; we have not been defeated. We speak out on behalf of right morals and strong values not because we fear death, but because we embrace life; we have not been defeated.

When newly infected members come hesitantly into our midst, terrified at their diagnosis, we show them that we have not been defeated. When those we love lie down to rest, and we must finally let them go, we celebrate their lives and all that they've given—they've merely died, as will we all. They have not been defeated.

And when someday my children come wandering alone through a crowd, seeking a word of comfort from the AIDS community, some reason for courage, one moment of your attention, you tell them, "She was not defeated, Max; she did not give in, Zack." Give them a hug, not for sympathy, but for strength. Show them that life has value that death cannot snatch. And— so they will not fear their own defeat in that hard moment— walk, if you can, a little way down the pilgrim road holding their hands.

Until that day, grace to you, and peace.

OFFERING THE CHILDREN

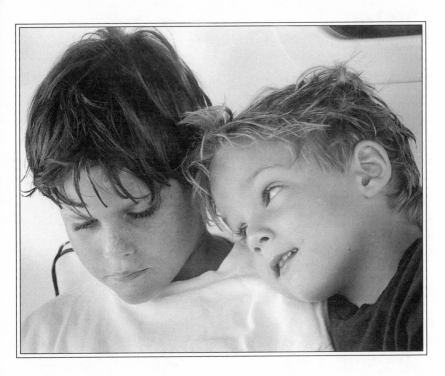

Victory of Spirit Award and Public Address
University of Louisville, School of Music Recital Hall
Louisville, Kentucky
Wednesday, October 19, 1994

———

The late Barry Bingham Sr. was a legendary publisher of the
Louisville Courier-Journal *during its heyday, which is still*
within memory. He was a man of great moral and profes-
sional elegance, more devoted to convictions than to cash flow.
He believed, passionately, that one should do what is right,
whether or not that is expedient.

In his honor, a Victory of Spirit Award is granted from time
to time by the University of Louisville and the Louisville Com-
munity Foundation, supported by a generous and anonymous
donation. The award is intended to spotlight ethical thought
and action, and to call for a publishable lecture by the award
recipient.

Robert Frost observed that there's something in us that dis-
likes fences. I discovered in Louisville (my birthplace, inciden-
tally) that there's also something in us that is troubled by
receiving an award for ethical choices. Soon after I was told of
my selection, I began to ask myself such questions as, "Well,

how ethical was I when . . .?" and "If they really *knew me,*
wouldn't they be surprised?"

By the time I arrived in Louisville, I was feeling more grat-
itude than guilt. I was pleased to be the first woman recipient
of this award, and happy to offer a perspective on "ethics in
the marketplace" (the original title of this speech).

With the Victory of Spirit Award comes the request to speak
briefly, here, today, on the theme of the award: ethical conduct.
And I'm honored by this invitation.

If you believe that ethics have fallen on hard times in America, you should move to Washington, D.C., where I live. We *talk*
about ethics all the time there. We have special investigators to
prowl through the lives of senators, and special counsel to re-
view the former lives of presidents. The Congress itself is
dressed up with ethics rules, ethics guidelines, and standing
committees on—what else?—ethics.

Skeptics view this as a tribute to how bad things have become. They recall Mark Twain's claim that "it could probably
be shown by facts and figures that there is no distinctly native
American criminal class, except Congress." They argue that
"we should no more have a committee on ethics than a committee on breathing"—since both breathing and behaving should
come naturally to our leaders.

The problem, of course, is that ethics don't provide the rules
by which our leaders are chosen in either government or business. Marketing does.

As we endure the fevered close of another election season,
last-minute comments of neck-and-neck candidates have
nearly nothing to do with ethics and nearly everything to do
with polls. "Tell them what they want to hear" is the rule of the

day. If you want to win, you appeal to marketplace instincts as consistently, and as compellingly, as possible.

And it's not politics alone. From the pricey sneakers we put on our children to assure their broad acceptance by fellow kindergartners, to the colleges we hope they will attend; few of us, as parents, place ethics above economics when preparing our children to run the race for popularity within their own groups.

Look around campus. See what we'll do for approval in fraternities and sororities where we market ourselves. In fact, what will we *not* do—if everyone agrees that it's approved, and we're convinced that we'll win approval for joining in? Neither the faculty room nor the boardroom is immune to the marketplace ethics that shape our decision making.

Mark Twain may have been right. He once described how gossip is elevated to the level of gospel by giving it a new label: "Its name is Public Opinion," he wrote. "It is held in reverence. It settles everything. Some think it is the voice of God."

And so we do. Women were dragged from their homes for hangings in Salem, Massachusetts, because public opinion said it was good and right. Slaves were branded and chained and sold at auction, as preachers explained each Sunday that it was God's will. We cannot remember history without seeing marketplace ethics at work.

Germany in the 1930s had been rocked by economic and international losses. It was a community hungry for nationalism, for an ethic which said that to be German was to be good—and to be anything less pure was to be evil. It was a short goose step from this nationalism to the ovens. Marketplace ethics at work.

Americans after World War II dreaded, above all else, the evils of "godless Communism." We were haunted by the idea that evil men, who could take from us our victory, lurked in the shadows of Hollywood and Washington. We demanded a search for things and people "un-American," giving rise to the campaign of intimidation now associated with the name McCarthy. Marketplace ethics at work.

If the 1948 presidential election is remembered for anything, it is the picture of a victorious President Truman smiling and pointing at the newspaper headline announcing his defeat at the hands of Thomas Dewey. And there was special delight in the moment because Dewey was, as David Halberstam described him, "a cold piece of work." He was small in stature and large in self-importance; "he struts sitting down," said one critic.

But throughout the 1948 campaign, in a nation hungry for anti-communism, Dewey refused to use the Communist-in-government issue as a political weapon. When he debated the critical issue of whether the American Communist Party should be outlawed, he opposed both his advisers and the polls by saying, "You can't shoot an idea with a gun." "If I'm going to lose," Dewey told his advisers, let me "lose on something I believe in."

He lost. And in the world of pollsters and political markets, Dewey is remembered as the butt of a great, national joke, for which Truman holding aloft the headline is the punch line.

I'm not here to resurrect Thomas Dewey's political image. But I am here to remember his regard for ethics, even when it cost some points in the polls. He may have been better at ethics than elections.

The danger of a marketplace ethic is, of course, that it's a house built on the shifting sands of public opinion. It asks not "What's right?" but, instead, "What's popular?" It's always subject to the latest fad and recent rumor. It blurs the line between conscience and constituents, between what I admire and my desire to be admired. And when, as Twain warned, we believe that our opinions are the voice of God, the distance between mass appeal and mob rule becomes terrifyingly short.

In the summer of 1991 I received a telephone call from my late husband, Brian, telling me he'd tested positive for the virus that causes AIDS. Another day not long after, on another telephone, I heard the news that I'd joined Brian on the road to AIDS.

I've always believed we have our lives to spend, to cash in for something of value. In a nation drenched in athletic clubs and health magazines, it's clear we're willing to spend lavishly to give our lives greater length. But sooner or later, most of us are called to the question "How will I give my life greater depth?" We come to a time of choosing.

In my own case, I asked veterans in the AIDS community how I might help. Most said, "Just tell your story." One particularly gritty woman told me bluntly, "This is an epidemic that's been waiting for someone who looks like you to speak out."

Many of those close to me worried about my speaking out. They saw the cost of trading privacy, which I cherish, for publicity, which I don't enjoy. They imagined the terrors that had—we later learned—kept Arthur Ashe from going public any sooner than he needed to. And one very special and very heroic person in my life, Betty Ford, said simply, "Once you have said it all in public, you can never again take it back as if it were private."

But let me be candid: It was not abstract ethics that motivated me as I wrestled with my choices. It was the reality of two children: Max, then three, and Zack, just one. It was not heroism that appealed to me, but motherhood. It drove my fears that I would need to give up my children too early, and it nourished my hope that I could leave both a model and a legacy marked not by shame, but by dignity and decency, perhaps even courage.

And so, in early 1992, in the city to which we had moved

from Louisville four decades earlier, my story was told in the *Detroit Free Press*. What I'd imagined as a back-section story was, instead, a front-page piece. Within hours, the truth of Betty Ford's warning was blazingly clear to all of us. And a few months later, I was in Houston speaking to the 1992 Republican National Convention.

I spoke in Houston for only thirteen minutes between waves of better-known people. But when the speech was over, Larry King was waiting. Morning papers from New York to San Francisco ran parts of the text, and the speech was reprinted in its entirety in the *Los Angeles Times* and, a day later, in the *London Times*. Thirteen minutes, and I was famous. I'd made no scientific breakthrough. I'd announced no cure. I'd merely stood up and asked people to consider being compassionate—a singularly uncreative idea with distinctively ancient roots.

What do you think made those thirteen minutes so shocking, so newsworthy, that every media outlet I'd ever heard of wanted time with me when it was over? Was it my lovely words? My brilliant syntax? I don't think so, and I hope you don't either.

What shocked America was that a married woman, in her early forties, with two nice children—a Republican, even, with work experience in TV and government—had AIDS. That's all. It wasn't what I said; it's what I represented. At the athletic club in Philadelphia or the bridge club in Kansas City, here was "one of us" instead of "one of them." What made me shocking wasn't my distinctiveness, but my commonness. I didn't fit the caricature drawn by American stereotypes. I didn't look like AIDS.

Which is to say, it was less the content of Mary Fisher's speech than the content of America's soul that made a few minutes in Houston newsworthy. It was the stereotype drawn by marketplace ethics that made my appearance surprising.

We don't hang Salem women for witchcraft in the 1990s. But if men are gay and sick and dying and dependent on our charity, they might find hanging a more genteel abuse. We don't trade slaves on the open market today, but we trade in a public opinion that reduces whole classes of people to something less than fully human.

For more than a decade, the politics of AIDS was reduced to the value of "the gay vote." The question was not how many artists and playwrights were sick or how many fathers and sons were dying—the question was, how many votes will it cost us to support them? And we are not done with this evil yet. Marketplace ethics are still at work.

The voice of public opinion tells us that nice people don't get AIDS. Men must be gay and engaging in unspeakable acts; women must be promiscuous or drug abusers, or both. Children with AIDS are "innocent victims" precisely because adults with AIDS are not. Physicians declined to treat, and morticians declined to embalm, those ravaged by the virus. Where the voice of public opinion sounds like the voice of God, preachers have claimed that God is using AIDS to accomplish his justice. To help God out, some believers have taken time to burn houses of those with AIDS. Here are marketplace ethics at work.

In this context, it was motherhood that lured me into speaking out. Because I saw the thin line between mass polls and mob justice—and that my children were at risk from both.

My concern was frankly selfish: in my dying hour I did not want my children wondering about the difference between public opinion and their mother's love. I do not want someone representing the voice of God telling them that their father's painful death was justified, and their mother "got what she deserved."

And so I spoke, and so I speak—less as a show of heroism than as an act of defiance against all attempts to define those of us with AIDS as morally depraved and socially deviant. I speak out for two reasons: Max, who is now seven, and Zachary, now five.

I truly do not know what it was, exactly, that motivated white Americans to hide slaves on stops along the Underground Railroad. Neither do I know why Dutch Calvinists risked their lives to hide Polish Jews. Religion was an important ingredient in the recipe for some courage. And I suppose that there was this: a person whose life was not at risk saw a person whose life was, and said, "It could be me." In that one moment of clear thought, someone realized—correctly—that we who are human are, all of us, one.

The division into "us" and "them" is deadly. It justifies slavery and it fills ovens with Jews. It enabled America to believe it had nothing to fear from AIDS because the majority is heterosexual and we, the majority, were convinced that this was a gay man's disease. Only when the virus began infecting the majority—people like "us" instead of "them"—did our conscience awaken.

Even today the consequences of homophobia mark the AIDS movement. Legislation is named not for one of the hundreds of thousands of gay men who have died, but for Ryan White, a charming young and heterosexual teenager. These are acceptable: Arthur Ashe, Elizabeth Glaser, Magic Johnson . . . and Mary Fisher. Public opinion has not yet fully accepted that there is no "they" within the human race; there is only a massive "we."

But, now and again, someone sees the truth. A man comes by who hears the cries of an Argentine child, imprisoned for her parents' politics, being tortured by her jailers; "It could be my child," he says, and he launches a crusade toward justice. Because he is gay, a man on campus is held down in the shower room and abused with a broom handle by a laughing football team; one of you rises up to say, "It could be my brother." In such moments, the spirit of ethics is no faint abstraction. It is a blindingly clear reality, a demanding plea that you must answer with, at least, your life.

For those who walk it, the road to AIDS grows long. The vigor with which we start our journey withers. We discover fellow travelers whom we love, and then we lose them, losing a part of ourselves as well. My children are too old to forget their final memories of their father, and too young to know how to understand their loss. And I, who hugged Brian as he drew his last breath, am really no wiser than they. And so we go, down the road together, often laughing, occasionally crying, sometimes very, very quiet.

And then I come here and see you. Some of you are young enough to have your whole lives before you; others of you, like me, have lived awhile. Whatever our age, when morning breaks again, we'll be called to make decisions—ethical decisions—about how to cash in the energy and time we have been given.

If any are looking for ethical models who might be worthy of imitation, do not look to me. I was dragged into this crusade kicking and screaming, wanting—desperately—not to play this role. But others came by choice: doctors who gave up practices with high profits to care for patients with low blood counts and no insurance; nurses who set aside stigma to give wasting men not only a vial of medicine, but a long hug of courageous affection; lovers and parents, sisters and friends, people who became caregivers when the court of public opinion ruled against any care at all—these are the heroes who should take home awards, and there are plenty of them today in Louisville.

I only wish you would join them. Go beyond the stigma and discrimination that have scarred this epidemic since first it was detected a decade and a half ago. Reckon with what it means that there are at least one, and perhaps two, million Americans already on the road to AIDS. Do not let cowards hide in silence, and do not join them. When you hear the stigma, stand up and be counted. When you see the discrimination, step forward and take action.

And when you see my children, get ready to take my place and take their hands.

I do not know how far I've already come down the road, or how long it stretches before me. But, unless there is a miracle, I know that Max will need someone to explain not only the loss of his father, but also the absence of his mother. Zack, who now wonders where to find his "Sniffy" at bedtime, will instead wonder who'll read him a story or tuck him in, give him a kiss or whisper, "Sleep with the angels." You can face these moments with dripping emotionalism; or you can face them squarely, head-on, with a gripping sense of values that enables you to step in when I have needed to lie down and rest.

Really, I did not come to offer you a lecture today, in return for the high honor of the Victory of Spirit Award. I came to offer you my children. And to ask that you show them the difference between common knowledge and uncommon insight, between conventional wisdom and unconventional courage, between marketplace ethics and genuine compassion. Truly, it is not that difficult.

And for any who would take my offer, I have an ancient prayer: grace to you, and peace.

I'LL
NOT GO QUIETLY

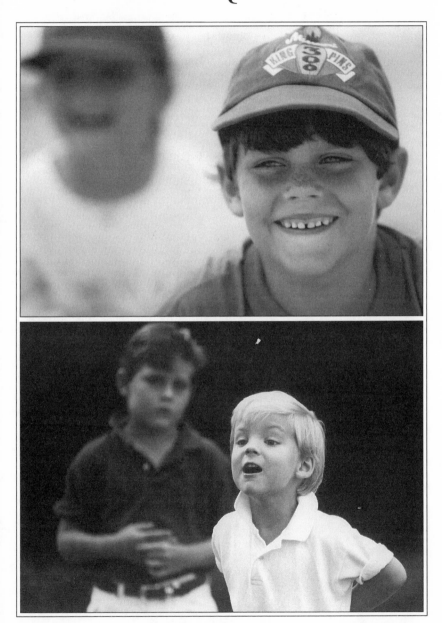

1994 National FFA Convention
Kansas City Convention Center
Kansas City, Missouri
Thursday, November 10, 1994

———

We had been in Kansas City in June as part of a local fund-raising effort, and to see family friends, Ambassador, (to the Court of St. James [England]) Charles and Carol Price. But this was a trip less to see Kansas City than to see the thirty-six thousand young people who had gathered to celebrate the FFA—what used to be the Future Farmers of America but is now simply "the FFA."

The event was held in Kemper Arena, where twelve thousand—a third of the convention crowd— of the cleanest, politest young Americans you've ever seen had just been entertained with a laser light show accompanied by exceedingly loud music. Then I was brought on to speak under a huge television screen on which a larger image of myself was visible even in the farthest reaches of the arena.

The appeal of this audience was obvious. Everywhere in America, we've chased the virus. It arrives first, begins devastating a community, and then—eventually—we begin our response. But here was an audience representing communities that have not yet been devastated. Here were thousands of young people who could be effectively warned and energetically invited to build compassionate communities.

It was a good place to find some fellow travelers for the days ahead, and to make the announcement: "With millions of others, I'll go down the road to AIDS—but I'll not go quietly."

I'm grateful to be here. What I have to say is not a speech I've given elsewhere. It will not be recycled in the months ahead. And neither, for what it's worth, is this a speech about being HIV-positive. It's an unvarnished appeal for you to become builders of community. And if it seems to you that this has nothing to do with AIDS, hear me out.

Margaret Mead, the great social anthropologist, told us that the best measure of a culture's character is how that culture treats its children. Remembering that, I want to tell you two stories.

Here is the first:

A young woman, planning a family Thanksgiving dinner, called her sister's home to make some quick, final arrangements. She was in a hurry—so when her four-year-old nephew answered, she skipped the usual playfulness and said, "Honey, let me talk to your mommy."

"She can't come to the phone right now," he whispered.

"Isn't she there?" she asked impatiently.

"She just can't come to the phone," he whispered.

"Well, then, let me talk to your daddy."

"He can't come to the phone right now."

"Well," she said, irritated, "is there anybody else there?"

"Yes." He was still whispering.

"Who?"

"The policeman and the fireman."

She knew it—her sister had always been so careless with the stove, and she'd warned her a hundred times. "Are you okay? What's everybody doing over there?"

"They're looking for me."

This story plays on a fundamental value of civilized society: its love for, and its fear of losing, its children. We worry about them because we love them. Your little brothers and sisters, your nephews and nieces, my sons, Max and Zack—we value our children above ourselves by instinct, by nature, by grace.

Which is why the second story was so hard to accept when it broke last week in Union, South Carolina. Distraught beyond reason, a young mother apparently strapped her two sons into the backseat of a car and sank it beneath the chilly waters of a nearby lake. After her boys drowned, she appealed for our help. She asked the nation to look for an abductor. And we were moved by her. Americans from coast to coast kept their eyes open for a car that was actually sitting at the bottom of a lake, containing two very small bodies.

The hour I learned I was HIV-positive, I grabbed for my children. I picked them up; I held them; I hugged them; I cried over them. I'm not a hero; I'm merely a mother, with motherly instincts.

And you—you are young adults, young enough to still be planning a future and adult enough to understand what the future may hold. And you are the first generation in history to come to adulthood in the context of AIDS. Fifteen years ago we thought only men in distant places were taken by this plague. We imagined that if we lived in the countryside or if we were women or if we maintained our conservative values, we would be saved from this scourge.

Now we know the truth. Having AIDS doesn't require being gay; it only requires being human, and being infected. Every state in the Union has been visited. Being rural or being Republican is no protection. And if we think either our gender or our age will protect us, we're mistaken: the epidemic is growing faster among women than among men, and fastest of all among adolescents.

Reports that the epidemic is fading are as reliable as the reports of an abduction in Union, South Carolina. The rate of deaths has slowed because so many of those initially infected have died; but the rates of infection are climbing while we speak, and the dying will pick up again in a year or two, because every one of us who is HIV-positive is a pilgrim on the road to AIDS.

The federal government says one million Americans are HIV-positive today; other reliable sources think, as I do, that the number is probably closer to two million. But let's take one million and give it perspective. The one million pilgrims on this road represent the combined total of every man, woman, and child in Fargo, North Dakota; Sioux City, Iowa; Sioux Falls, South Dakota; Cheyenne, Wyoming; Missoula, Montana; Lawrence, Kansas—and Minneapolis, Minnesota. At least, this was the size of the AIDS pilgrim band when you and I met a few moments ago; it's already grown larger while we've been together.

The question is: What are we going to do about it?

What I'm going to do is speak out. I understand what it means to be HIV-positive, because I'm fighting the disease every day. And I understand what it means to die of AIDS. I was with my late husband until an hour after he died. I helped my children say good-bye to their father. Now they walk with me, on the road to AIDS, wondering about another good-bye somewhere in the distance. As we walk, I speak out.

The larger question—twelve thousand times larger, at least—is: What do you intend to do? When a million or more pilgrims come down the road past America's farmlands, near your home, and one of us stops to ask for comfort, what are you going to say? When one of the pilgrims asks whether her life is as important as the price of soybeans, whether his future matters as much as the futures market in corn—how are you going to respond? Or, to put an edge on the question: When I am gone and my children ask you about me, what do you intend to say to them?

You might tell those passing by in the AIDS pilgrim band that you have learned from us. Give my life meaning by letting me know that, in seeing what I will suffer, you've learned to avoid the virus yourself. Let those who are HIV-positive be what we can be: warnings.

The cause of this disease is a virus that can only be passed from human to human through bodily fluids. You can't get it from a sneeze or hug; you don't get it by sharing a Coke or a secret. You get it by exchanging blood or semen or vaginal fluids or a mother's breast milk. This means that if you are sexually active, you should be sexually responsible: protect yourself. And if you've been sexually active and didn't protect yourself, then get tested. With a million carriers of this virus in America's adult population, no one who's had unprotected sex can say that they are safe.

So this is the first appeal I make to you: learn from those of us who learned too late. Don't take chances with your life or the lives of those you say you love. Be responsible.

A second appeal is aimed directly to those of you who are planning careers in agriculture. I want you to teach America something about death.

Those who know agriculture know that death is as ordinary as birth, and as miraculous. Unless the seed falls to the ground and perishes, there is no golden wheat. Until the kernel gives up its life to nourish the corn, our fields are dark and barren.

The newborn calf struggles to its feet as the old cattle lie down to die. Those whose livelihood is planted in the soil understand death far better than those who are insulated from it.

The million or so pilgrims on the road to AIDS talk about death often, because it travels with us. It's as natural for us as for a family farmer who points toward the graves on a nearby hillside and talks of those who first cut the sod or stacked the stones. And it's important that you talk back. Don't be afraid of those of us who are dying. We merely wonder if we will be alone the hour we die, if we will be put away where no one will talk to us or listen to us or pray with us.

You who are planting your careers in the life-and-death cycle of agriculture know that death is as real as life. You have to know that, or you will fail. All that I'm asking is that you act on that knowledge by reaching out fearlessly to those infected with the AIDS virus. That's all.

Hearing that request, you've already heard my final appeal: I want you to go home from Kansas City convinced of the need to build community.

I am of your parents' generation. We've not done very well at building community. We are giving you a nation torn apart by our generation and those that came before us: North against South, white against black, resident against immigrant, straight against gay, Republican against Democrat, urban against rural. We've cared more for the value of our private property than the values of our public community. We've protected our assets more than our children. And, in the end, it is the children who will pay.

A powerful lesson was delivered late last weekend in a newscast from Union, South Carolina. A citizen of that town was asked how he felt about the tragedy. He looked away from the camera for a moment, and then down; he shifted from foot to foot; and then, in a drawl as warm as a Carolina morning, he said, "I'm ashamed for my community's name."

Drug dealers break bones of children to get more cash from their parents; the landlord worries about his rent, but doesn't feel ashamed of his community. A man breaks into our local post office and kills colleagues; we thank God that we were spared, but we don't feel embarrassment that it was our post office. Children with AIDS are told not to enroll in school; men with AIDS are told not to come to work; women with AIDS are told they don't deserve to keep their children—and no one says, "We're ashamed."

I'm not a fan of shame, but I love community. And when we can no longer feel shame for our community, it's probably because there's no community left for which to feel anything at all.

America didn't respond to AIDS in the beginning because we lacked community with those who were gay. We hate to say it, but our behaviors prove it: we did not care if gay men died. Until AIDS knocked on our door, we said, "Let those who are careless pay for their own carelessness." While the numbers of the infected grew, we thanked God it was them, not us. We made a mockery of our faith and of our compassion and of any claim to have community.

The essence of community is this: we are bound together, we are one. You have no suffering I do not bear. When farmers fight first floods and then a blight, it is my fight in which they are engaged. And when I fight for my life against a deadly virus, it is—or is it?—your fight as well.

You have ambition, or you would not be here. You have commitment to a career and an agricultural tradition that is deep and rich. I salute that tradition, and I congratulate you for it.

But if your ambition is purely personal; if your sole measures of success are bank accounts and acreage charts—I do not wish you well. I wish you, instead, better wisdom.

Here's what better wisdom looks like: Find a child whose mother is on the edge of panic and hold that child safely—lest the sound of a seat belt's snapping shut make all of us, again, shake our heads in sad amazement. Find a woman who's abandoned hope that the dirt will ever give up a crop, that her husband will ever tell her, again, that he loves her—and reach out for her in comfort, before she becomes yet another casualty of yet another, quiet farmhouse death.

There's a little boy who's desperate for his older brother to say one kind word to him; you're the older brother. There's a little girl who's ready to imitate the worst example you ever set, because you told her it was cool; go home and change her mind. It doesn't take miracles; it takes integrity. From raking leaves for an aging widow to shoveling snow for an irritated neighbor—there are thousands of ways to build community, and none of them require much more than a simple, single act of kindness.

We've worried too long and too hard about building bank accounts. And we've worried too late and too little about building communities strong enough to hold those who are weak, courageous enough to defend those who are struggling, and compassionate enough to whisper a sweet good-bye to those at death's doorstep.

We need to build community, and we need you to do it. You're gifted adults still young enough to change your entire lives. You're ready to give a liberal dose of ambition to a career shaped by conservative values. There is no other audience like you in the world.

And I'm eager to speak to you because I'm not on some liberal crusade: I'm merely on the road to AIDS. Bending over the bed of one who's out ahead of me on this road, I can sometimes feel death. I count the beats of their pulse and wonder how many days I have left. I hear their stories and wonder how my own will end. I remember carrying Max and Zack from their father's grave and wonder who will carry them from mine. I grow melancholy, and a little discouraged. I think maybe I should give it up, pack it in.

And then I hear a seven-year-old hollering up the stairs, "Mom, the dog did it in the kitchen again!" A five-year-old flies into my bedroom with a crayon masterpiece he made for me at school. Grim thoughts about death are drenched with everyday life. I turn from the agony of the road to AIDS and feel the ecstasy of my own children. And I take, again, this single vow: with millions of others, I'll go down the road to AIDS—but I'll not go quietly.

And I do not want to go alone. I want, desperately, for you to come with me. You may not be able to hand me a cure, but you could walk with me and tell some pilgrim woman that she's worth the effort it takes to build community. You may not be able to save his life, but you could turn to a gay man whose family says he does not matter and prove to him that God has better messages to bring than judgment. You could protect yourself and then turn to build community. Come with me to tell people we pass that the pilgrims who are sick need healing, not discrimination; they need compassion, not rejection; comfort, not condemnation.

You've come to Kansas City, as have I. And soon we'll go home again. Don't go quietly. Let my children hear you calling for a community in which we would be ashamed, not of having AIDS, but of rejecting those who have it. Let the children you love see a model not of discrimination, but of affection, which binds together broken communities and heals us of our own diseases.

Come, build community with me along the road to AIDS.

Take the hands of Max and Zack and show them courage. Be ready to go on without me; but do not go on without them. Hold them tightly, cuddle them with community, and listen closely— and no matter how far you've gone, you'll still hear me say in gratitude to God and you: grace to you, and peace.

Closing
daddy's diary

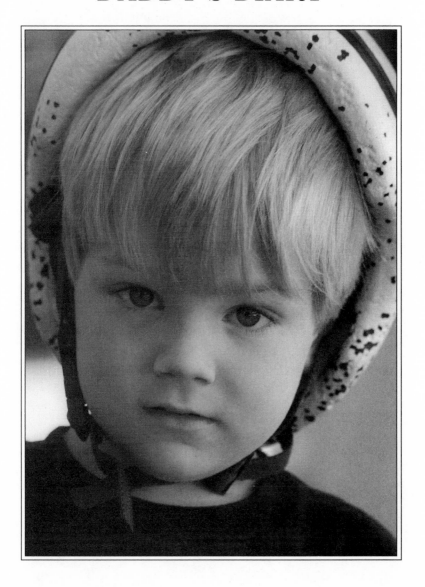

American Jewish Committee Tribute to Max M. Fisher
New York City
Sunday, December 4, 1994

———

I knew, before I gave this speech, that it would be the last entry in this book. We would open with the memorial for Brian, who had died before his children had both cleared kindergarten; we would close with a tribute to my father, offered in his eighty-sixth year.

The road between Brian's memorial and my father's tribute took some surprising turns. Many of the most joyful surprises were people. Annie and Greg Willard rescued me from a lonesome trip by filling my time with joy. John Burkoff first invited me to Pittsburgh and then honored me with his constant presence, assuring me that the story I told had value. On more than one occasion, Rosie O'Donnell slipped in, showing in her eyes a tender and generous soul sometimes overlooked by those who laugh hardest at her routines. And there's Judith Light, a saint who masquerades as an actress. Each of them, and others, have made it possible for me to stand again, be vulnerable again, tell the story one more time.

The story of AIDS in America is told in a glance at these bookend speeches. We are giving up much of the nation's "middle generation"—millions of people of child-rearing age who will become patients, then statistics, then casualties, but never grandparents.

The epidemic never touches a stranger. It always, only, takes members of families. It claims people on whom others had a prior claim: husbands who had been promised to their wives, children who were not ready to let go of their mother.

And so I rose to pay tribute to my father. I spoke as a daughter, not an AIDS community representative. But the distinction is terribly thin. Because the AIDS community is made up exclusively of people like me. Mothers and fathers who want not to let go of their children. Brothers and sisters who cling to each other, desperate for strength. Sons and daughters who are eager to tell their father that they love him, hopeful that they will hear back, "And I love you."

My father is not a man who appreciates public displays of emotion, and I wasn't sure how he'd react to having one of his children stand up and speak about him as "Daddy."

I asked my mother what she thought and she said, in her typically genteel way, "Don't worry about it; he usually falls asleep by seven-thirty anyway. Just keep it short, will you, Mary?"

Some of you may know that my father's professional discretion and public decorum have been balanced for the past four decades by my mother's personal habits and private humor. It isn't true, as some friends have alleged, that they are a comedy team in which he plays the straight man. But it is true that they are, together, a remarkable balance of chaos and order.

Bill Moyers, who went from being a Baptist preacher to being Lyndon Johnson's press secretary, tells the story of a weekend visit to the LBJ ranch during Johnson's presidency. On Sunday noon lunch was served outdoors on an enormous table seating more than one hundred guests, with the president at one end and his press secretary at the other. As everyone took their seats, Johnson roared down the table, "Moyers, say grace." Dutifully, Moyers stood and began offering a suitably ecumenical blessing. Midway through it, the president bellowed out, "Moyers, I can't hear you!" And Moyers responded, "Actually, Mr. President, I wasn't speaking to you."

I tell you this story as background to the following belief, widely held within our family. People account for my father's longevity and vitality in a variety of ways. Our family is convinced that, although God may have tried to call my father home, Daddy didn't approve the idea. And that was that.

I understand this is the second occasion on which you've conferred the National Distinguished Leadership Award in its present format. On behalf of my sisters, my brother, my mother, and all of our family, I want to thank you for this year's selection.

One reason we're grateful, of course, is that we love the man you've chosen. As a mother, I take enormous joy in seeing others praise my children. But, especially as the years have moved by, I've taken a similar pleasure—as have all of us in the family—in seeing Daddy's accomplishments recognized.

My father has long held that "there is no such thing as a devil or a saint." I've never heard him speak of himself in saintly terms, although one or the other of us children may have tempted him to reconsider his position on devils.

Those of you here this evening know something of the history of the American Jewry. You know the divisions that have sometimes formed, the positions that have torn at us. You know the struggle that's been required to unite us on critical issues, and the reality that we have not always been united. And therefore you know that Max Fisher has not always been seen as the patron saint of this cause.

We are, as a family, grateful that you chose to offer Daddy a warm tribute tonight, rather than a moving eulogy at some point down the road. And we are pleased for the most obvious of all reasons: he is here to see and hear it.

And we're pleased because of a truth many of you may not know—or may not believe: what will please him about this event is not that he will have been praised as a saintly Jewish leader, but that his selection is another evidence of Jewish unity.

My father has been committed, sometimes to the edge of obsession, to the goal of unity. And he has given to this cause until it nearly broke his heart.

On January 1, 1973, my father took pen in hand and wrote an extraordinary entry into his private diary. He had spent himself in years of pursuing Israel's welfare. And, on that New Year's morning, he assessed the cost: "I have lost a great deal," he wrote. "No one can really appreciate what I have lost except myself." He was desperate to reestablish, as he put it, a "relationship to my family." Without it, he wrote, "this is something I will suffer from more than anything else."

On behalf of those who shared his sacrifice, thank you for telling my father, on this evening and in this way, that the cost was worth it.

Second, I would like to speak briefly to all of us, me and my family included, not as representatives of a cause but as individuals.

If a clever Palestinian decided to exchange peace for war, blowing up this room would remove a good deal of the leadership of the American Jewish community in a blazing moment.

You are a potent force in this nation, both within and beyond the Jewish community. You've created corporations and nurtured them, defined policies and pursued them, identified candidates and elected them. You've achieved more than any Jewish mother had a right to imagine—or any Jewish father would ever believe, no matter what evidence you presented. We'll not help ourselves by engaging in hours of self-congratulation. But neither will we help others by engaging in denial of the power that we hold. My appeal to you this evening is to use the power you have to create a more compassionate national community.

The Committee has a proud history of defending civil and individual rights. From the amicus brief that helped weaken the grip of the Ku Klux Klan in the Pacific Northwest to our role in *Brown versus the Board of Education*—the AJC has forged a record worthy of emulation. We have championed the ideal of an American community.

My father has distinguished himself, and imprinted his family, with this same value. He has taken up causes because he absolutely believes the community has *earned* his contribution. Philanthropy is not something he merely does; it is something he believes is a repayment.

We remember his pledges to Israel; but we would also do well to remember that he grieved with special grief not only for the crumbling walls of Jerusalem, but for the burning city of Detroit. His commitment to racial justice and human dignity has been so pervasive in my lifetime that when I first encountered genuine prejudice as an adult, I did not know what it was.

My wish this evening for myself, and for all like me, is that we honor my father not merely with tributes but with imitation. The American community has been whipped with injustice and battered by prejudice. Long after laws prohibited segregation in the voting booth, our corporate offices remain largely segre-

gated. Those who are African-American or Caribbean or His-
panic—all have been given reason to ask, "Where do we find
true community?" Those who are immigrants, who are poor,
who are wasting from incurable diseases—all wonder if community is designed to invite them in for the holidays or to shut
them out at the gate of privilege, and we give them reason to
wonder. I know gay men with AIDS who can explain with great
clarity the short supply of compassion in this world.

To honor my father, we need not sing his praises; but we do
need to pursue his passion for community. We cannot do this
without embracing compassion. If we do not, what we are offering this evening is not honor at all; it is hypocrisy.

And, finally, this is a glorious occasion for me because I have
the podium and my father has no choice but to listen. For forty-
six years I've hungered and thirsted after such a moment. And I
don't intend to pass it by without saying what he might otherwise not hear.

I think, Daddy, that you are still with us, not because you've
refused God's desire to take you, but because you've been faith-
ful to your calling. And he's not done with you, here, yet.

There is still work to do in the professional world, where corporate leaders seek your counsel because they know you have
not only power, which is relatively common, but wisdom, which
is terribly rare.

There is still work to do in the philanthropic world, where it's
not only your money that is treasured but your vision. It is the
Treasury that mints money, but the origin of your vision is in the
prophets who saw a kingdom not yet built and called for its cre-
ation. It's your vision that's needed most.

There is still work to do in politics, and in various Jewish
causes. There is work that will never be completed.

But when you turn away from your work, you will hear your

family telling God we're glad you are still here—for us. No matter what you wrote on that distant New Year's morning, you have not lost us. It is not our loss that you suffer, Daddy. It is our presence. We ain't been easy, and we still aren't.

You worry that we're going to spend you into poverty, and you warn us about it. You worry that we're going to make rash decisions, and you warn us against them. You worry that the family won't hold together, that we'll come apart like many others you've seen.

Your family is going to hold together, Daddy. It isn't your checkbook that brings us home; it's the hope that we will hear you say you are proud of what we're doing. It isn't your reputation that holds us in your sway; it's our conviction that, without you, we would be less than we are today.

Tributes come and tributes go. But the counsel of Henry Wadsworth Longfellow endures:

> Not in the clamor of the crowded street,
> Not in the shouts and plaudits of the throng,
> But in ourselves, are triumph and defeat.
>
> —"The Poets"

In you, Daddy, we have learned something of the cost of both triumph and defeat. Above all else, we've learned that integrity outlasts both of them—and that integrity is found within ourselves, often in the meanest hour of the night.

Peter Golden captured in his biography of you the sometimes cold spirit of your father, Daddy, and used that spirit as the backdrop to what may be the single most tender moment in the narrative.

It was January 1971. You were in Israel with my brother, Phillip, when word came that your father had died. A few days later, standing with my cousin Sherry by his coffin, you reached out and stroked your father's hair. After a moment, you said to Sherry, "Dad always liked that."

It is not clear, Daddy, whether I will stroke your hair someday, or you will stroke mine. I do not enjoy being on the road to AIDS very much, and you do not enjoy being unable to change that. But, in the end, it will not matter. Because, here and now, we can do something much finer than stroke hair. We can still lean over at a banquet table and whisper, "I love you." Jane and Margie, Julie and Phillip, Mom and I—we've always liked that.

Those of us who've come to pay you honor may go home tonight to seek new ways to build community, to show compassion, to pursue justice.

And when you go home tonight, Daddy, you may rip up the New Year's diary from 1973. Replace it with this evening's tribute. Hear the sound of public applause. But go to sleep feeling Mom's fingers running through your hair, and hearing one of the children whisper, "Daddy, I love you." Good night.

NOTEBOOK

From the adjournment of the National Commission on AIDS—June 28, 1993—through the winter holidays of 1994, we crisscrossed the nation, speaking to diverse groups in sometimes surprising settings. Variations of excerpts published in this book were sometimes included in addresses to other groups as well.

Ocala, Florida, Ocala Public High School, Friday, September 10, 1993

Ocala, Florida, Ed Keeton Memorial Lecture Series, Friday, September 10, 1993

Birmingham, Alabama, Vestavia Hills United Methodist Church, Sunday, September 12, 1993

Birmingham, Alabama, Sixteenth Street Baptist Church, Sunday, September 12, 1993

Birmingham, Alabama, Jewish Federation Physicians Dinner, Sunday, September 12, 1993

Birmingham, Alabama, Temple Emmanuel, Sunday, September 12, 1993

Birmingham, Alabama, Community-Based AIDS Organizations, Sunday, September 12, 1993

Birmingham, Alabama, Clergy AIDS Education Project, Monday, September 13, 1993

Washington, D.C., AIDS Walk Washington, Saturday, September 18, 1993

Atlantic City, New Jersey, Miss America Pageant, Saturday,
September 18, 1993

Madison, Wisconsin, Wisconsin HIV/AIDS Program Conference, Monday, September 20, 1993

Provincetown, Massachusetts, Brian Campbell Memorial Service, Saturday, September 25, 1993

San Juan, Puerto Rico, Special Session of the Senate, Tuesday,
September 28, 1993

San Juan, Puerto Rico, Chamber of Commerce HIV/AIDS Symposium, Tuesday, September 28, 1993

Bloomfield Hills, Michigan, Cranbrook Educational Community Founder's Award Dinner, Saturday, October 2, 1993

Salt Lake City, Utah, AIDS Memorial Quilt Opening Ceremony,
Thursday, October 14, 1993

Salt Lake City, Utah, National Hospice Organization Annual
Symposium and Exposition Opening Address, Friday,
October 15, 1993

Houston, Texas, Opening Ceremonies for the NAMES Project
AIDS Memorial Quilt, Sunday, October 17, 1993

Houston, Texas, HIV/AIDS Service Providers Breakfast, Monday, October 18, 1993

Nashville, Tennessee, Vanderbilt University Forum, Tuesday,
October 19, 1993

Grand Rapids, Michigan, Council of Michigan Foundations,
Friday, November 5, 1993

Los Angeles, California, First AME Church of Los Angeles,
Sunday, November 14, 1993

Rancho Mirage, California, Betty Ford Center, Monday,
November 15, 1993

Los Angeles, California, UCLA Board of Visitors, Tuesday,
November 16, 1993

Los Angeles, California USC Public Forum, Tuesday,
November 16, 1993

Atlanta, Georgia, Cascade United Methodist Church, Sunday, November 21, 1993

Atlanta, Georgia, Atlanta AIDS Interfaith Hope & Healing Service, Sunday, November 21, 1993

Atlanta, Georgia, Paideia Private School—Junior and Senior High, Monday, November 22, 1993

New York City, Jeffrey Schmalz Memorial Service, Tuesday, December 7, 1993

New York City, STEP Program at Riker's Island, Tuesday, December 7, 1993

Washington, D.C., International Skye Working Group of Families, Wednesday, December 8, 1993

Lansing, Michigan, Michigan State University Commencement, Saturday, December 11, 1993

Miami Beach, Florida, University of Miami School of Medicine ANTRA Award Dinner, Saturday, December 11, 1993

Rancho Mirage, California, Betty Ford Center, Monday, February 21, 1994

Greenwich, Connecticut, Greenwich Academy, Thursday, March 10, 1994

New York City, Riker's Island STEP Program Commencement Address, Friday, March 11, 1994

Dallas, Texas, National United Way Conference, Monday, March 21, 1994

Santa Fe, New Mexico, Northern New Mexico AIDS Center, Wednesday, April 20, 1994

Pittsburgh, Pennsylvania, Temple Sinai, Sunday, April 24, 1994

Pittsburgh, Pennsylvania, Taylor Alderdice High School, Monday, April 25, 1994

Pittsburgh, Pennsylvania, University of Pittsburgh School of Law, Monday, April 25, 1994

Rock Island, Illinois, Augustana College, Tuesday, May 3, 1994

Moline, Illinois, Moline High School, Wednesday, May 4, 1994

Toronto, Ontario, Canada, CANFAR Breakfast for Attorneys, Monday, May 9, 1994

Toronto, Ontario, Canada, 1994 Unique Lives & Experiences Lecture Series, Monday, May 9, 1994

San Francisco, California, San Francisco AIDS Foundation Leadership Dinner, Tuesday, May 10, 1994

New York City, Sotheby's, Wednesday, June 8, 1994

East Meadow, New York, Fifth Annual HIV for the Non-Infectious Disease Physician Symposium, Thursday, June 9, 1994

Kansas City, Missouri, St. Paul's Episcopal Church, Thursday, June 16, 1994

Kansas City, Missouri, AIDS Ribbon of Hope Benefit Dinner, Thursday, June 16, 1994

Kansas City, Missouri, AIDS Network Service Providers, Friday, June 17, 1994

Washington, D.C., FDA Blood Products Advisory Committee Hearing on Home-Access HIV Testing, Wednesday, June 22, 1994

Durham, North Carolina, Duke University Continuing Medical Education Conference, Saturday, June 25, 1994

Washington, D.C., Congress on Women's Health, Tuesday, June 28, 1994

St. Louis, Missouri, Missouri/Illinois HIV/AIDS Network Educational Conference, Friday, July 22, 1994

San Francisco, California, Baseball Chapels for SF Giants and Colorado Rockies, Sunday, July 31, 1994

San Francisco, California, Candlestick Park, "Until There's a Cure Day" Giants Baseball Game, Sunday, July 31, 1994

San Francisco, California, Project Open Hand, Monday, August 1, 1994

Pontiac, Michigan, Lomas Brown Foundation Dinner, Tuesday, September 27, 1994

Montgomery, Alabama, AIDS Task Force of Alabama Annual Awards Dinner, Thursday, October 6, 1994

Montgomery, Alabama, Alabama AIDS Symposium, Friday, October 7, 1994

Montgomery, Alabama, Jefferson Davis High School, Friday, October 7, 1994

Brooklyn, New York, New York City Obstetricians and Gynecologists Luncheon, Friday, October 14, 1994

Louisville, Kentucky, Victory of Spirit Award and Public Address, University of Louisville, School of Music Recital Hall, Wednesday, October 19, 1994

Louisville, Kentucky, University of Louisville, Thursday, October 20, 1994

Boston, Massachusetts, Boston College, Thursday, October 27, 1994

Boston, Massachusetts, Benefit Luncheon for Rosie's Place, Friday, October 28, 1994

Boston, Massachusetts, American Association of Medical Colleges, Saturday, October 29, 1994

Bethesda, Maryland, Burning Tree Elementary School PTA, Tuesday, November 1, 1994

Kansas City, Missouri, 1994 National FFA Convention, Thursday, November 10, 1994

Toms River, New Jersey, Toms River Presbyterian Church, Sunday, December 4, 1994

New York City, American Jewish Committee Tribute to Max M. Fisher, Sunday, December 4, 1994

INDEX

*Page numbers printed in **boldface** indicate photographs*